NUTRITION AND DIET RESEARCH PROGRESS

VEGETABLE CONSUMPTION AND HEALTH:

NEW RESEARCH

Nutrition and Diet Research Progress

Additional books in this series can be found on Nova's website
under the Series tab.

Additional E-books in this series can be found on Nova's website
under the E-book tab.

Food and Beverage Consumption and Health

Additional books in this series can be found on Nova's website
under the Series tab.

Additional E-books in this series can be found on Nova's website
under the E-book tab.

NUTRITION AND DIET RESEARCH PROGRESS

VEGETABLE CONSUMPTION AND HEALTH:

NEW RESEARCH

CLAUDIA WILSON
AND
MELINDA MORREE
EDITORS

Nova Science Publishers, Inc.
New York

LIBRARY OF CONGRESS CATALOGING-IN-PUBLICATION DATA

Vegetable consumption and health : new research / editors, Claudia Wilson and Melinda Morree.
p. ; cm.
Includes bibliographical references and index.
ISBN 978-1-62100-941-2 (hardcover)
I. Wilson, Claudia, 1971 Mar. 26- II. Morree, Melinda.
[DNLM: 1. Nutrition Therapy. 2. Vegetables. 3. Nutritive Value. WB 430]

615.8'54--dc23

2011040544

Published by Nova Science Publishers, Inc. + New York

CONTENTS

PREFACE

It is well-known that diets high in vegetables are associated with lower rates of chronic diseases and cancers. Vegetables provide a good source of nutrients and dietary fiber which are essential for various bodily functions. Throughout the world, though, reported vegetable consumption is well below the recommended levels set by the World Health Organization. In this book, the authors present current research in the study of vegetable consumption and health. Topics discussed include food insecurity and vegetable consumption; quality control for pesticide residues in olives and olive oil; pest management of cruciferous crops in China; availability and utilization of traditional vegetables; cucumbers as a source of biological active substances and vegetable consumption by older adults in Japan.

Chapter 1 - Over 14.7% of U.S. households experienced food insecurity in 2009, while 21.3% of households with children under 18 and 22.9% of households with children under six were food insecure. In about 40% of food insecure households, one or more family members has experienced disruptions in normal eating patterns and reduced food intake due to limited resources. Low-income households are, unsurprisingly, less likely to purchase vegetables due to cost and availability and more likely to purchase affordable, energy-dense, nutrient-poor foods, which contain refined carbohydrates, added fats, and added sugars. Despite the availability of low-cost vegetable options in many communities, low-income mothers responsible for food purchasing and preparation perceive cost as a substantial barrier to vegetable consumption. Food insecurity may exacerbate some of the worrisome shopping and food consumption patterns observed in low-income households. One recent study of Latino households showed that household food insecurity was associated with lower quantities and less variety of fruits and vegetables in the home. Food insecurity is also related to decreased consumption of fruits and vegetables among adults as household resources deplete. Some studies have shown links between food insecurity and poor behavioral and academic outcomes for children, while other studies identified connections between parental psychological distress, family dysfunction, and low parent and child vegetable consumption. While few studies have attempted to parse out the causal pathway linking these various factors, it is possible that the stressful experiences and limited choices associated with poverty and food security undermine parents' abilities to access, afford, and provide healthful foods in the context of limited resources. Literature linking food insecurity with low vegetable consumption, however, is inconclusive, underscoring the need for improvements in study design to examine causal relationships between poverty, food insecurity, and vegetable consumption. In this chapter, the authors review the current state of knowledge on the indeterminate relationship between food security status and vegetable consumption, addressing the role of culture, the importance of safety net programs, and methodological issues.

Chapter 2 - Olive oil is a product of great importance in the sustainable economy of important regions from the main olive oil producers in the world, Spain, Italy and Greece. Due to the facts that virgin olive oil production has increased in recent years and that it is being exported to different countries, exhaustive quality controls are required. The application of phytosanitary products is one of the main employed procedures to solve the problems of plagues and diseases in olive groves. As a result, there is an increasing unease related to the possible presence of residues from these products in the olive-derived foods. Recent studies have shown that these residues can be found in olives and olive oil (mainly insecticides, fungicides and herbicides) due to the lipophilic nature of the used plaguicides. Different regulations regarding maximum residue limits (MRLs) in table olives and olive oil have been established by the European Union and the Codex Alimentarius of the Food and Agriculture Organization of the United Nations; in addition, new regulations will be established in following years. However, the detected levels of all these phytosanitary products are usually below the MRLs established. A wide range of pesticides is used by olive farmers for pest management and vector control in agricultural areas. Sometimes, farmers use these compounds without full understanding of their impact on human health and the environment. Although the inhalation, dermal and oral routes of exposure are the most common, pesticide residues in food and water may add to indirect exposures in the general population. This constitutes a risk of these pesticides being incorporated in both: (a) rivers and reservoirs with the soil that is eroded in heavy rains, polluting surface waters, etc.; and (b) olives and, consequently, olive oil. There are alternative methods available for the analysis of pesticides in different kind of samples. However, the common methods of analysis for their determination are Gas Chromatography (GC) and Liquid Chromatography (LC). GC is usually the chosen technique due to the high separation efficiency and compatibility with a wide range of detection techniques.The authors' research group has performed thorough investigation over the analysis of pesticides in soils, olive fruits and virgin olive oils. In particular, the authors have developed different GC analytical methods with mass spectrometric detection for the analysis of all the main pesticides used in olive groves. In this way, sensitive and reliable procedures can be implemented for the quality control of table olives and olive oils in the industry. These methodologies will be briefly described in this chapter.

Chapter 3 - The advent of photosynthesis is one of the central events in the early development of life on Earth. The origin and evolution of photosynthesis, however, has long remained unresolved. Any studious individual who wishes to appreciate the big picture of how photosynthesis works and how it fits into the broad scope of scientific inquiry needs to have at least a rudimentary understanding of numerous fields of science. This is an increasingly difficult task in this age of scientific specialization, because no one can truly be an expert in all areas. The intent of this paper is not to advance knowledge on the plant process presently called photosynthesis, a very important photochemical process considered to be the origin of the food chain that is still not yet completely understood in spite of the fact it has already seen 350 years of study. Rather, this article attempts to provide a starting point for an unsuspected metabolic pathway over and above what we know about plants, the hitherto unknown capability of Melanin, the animal analogue to Chlorophyll, to harvest electromagnetic radiations to use as energy to dissociate the water molecule with a subsequent release of energy. An analogue process with that of plants, so similar in animal cells to the first step in plant photosynthesis (absorption of light/dissociation of water), that the authors have named it "Human Photosynthesis."

Chapter 4 - Cruciferous vegetables are one of the dominant food crops, and widely considered to be healthy foods containing multiple nutrients and phytochemicals. In China, cruciferous crops are mainly infested by lepidopteran, coleopteran and hemipteran pests, causing damage through the loss of crop yield or quality. Pest control has relied heavily on the application of chemical pesticides for a long time but many problems are associated with their use such as the appearance of resistant strains of pests and harmful effects on non-target organisms. To achieve better control of pests in cruciferous crops, efforts since the 1990s have been focused on developing and implementing integrated pest management (IPM) incorporating various environmentally benign approaches, including cultural practices, conservation biological control and behavioral regulation. The IPM system was designed as a flexible framework to minimize adverse effects on vegetable products, non-target species and environment, to maximize profit for growers, and to be sustainable. Over the past two decades, this IPM program has been extensively used to effectively control the major insect pests in cruciferous crops in the southern provinces of China, and proved to be ecologically sound, economically feasible, environmentally acceptable, and practically applicable.

Chapter 5 - Micronutrient deficiency is a major challenge in resource poor households of South Africa. While traditional vegetables have been identified as one of the strategies to alleviate micronutrient deficiency in such households, research has shown a decline in the use of traditional vegetables in favour of introduced vegetables. Traditional vegetables, unlike introduced vegetables, can survive poor soil, require less agricultural inputs and resources during production and are often available at times when introduced vegetables are scarce. Knowledge about traditional vegetables is vanishing due to the decline in traditional vegetable use. Since documentation of traditional vegetables is scarce, elderly people remain the most valuable source of knowledge. Due to a general reluctance of the youth to gain knowledge associated with the utilisation of traditional vegetables, the fear exist that valuable indigenous knowledge on traditional vegetables might disappear completely from society. Research was conducted to determine the availability of traditional vegetables at eMantlaneni village close to Lusikisiki in the Eastern Cape Province of South Africa. The extent of traditional vegetable use was determined and the collection, storage, preservation and cooking practices of traditional vegetables were documented. The larger significance of the research not only lies in the documentation of the associated indigenous knowledge that is in danger of being lost, but also in establishing utilisation patterns that can be used to compare regional variations in collection, storage, cooking and preservation practices. The study envisioned that more knowledge about traditional vegetables could improve food diversity which will translate to the improvement of nutritional status of resource poor households. The research was limited to a single case study, documenting the practices of one South African cultural grouping (Xhosa cultural practices). The study could also not include the nutritional value of the traditional vegetables, although this has been identified as need for further research. Main findings of the research showed that thirty three traditional vegetables were identified and their collection, storage, preservation and cooking practices were described. Already accessibility to some traditional vegetables poses a problem due to women having to travel long distances to gather these scarce traditional vegetables. The study concluded that the suitability of traditional vegetables rests on their benefits of being readily available, low agricultural input and reported nutritional value. Because of these benefits traditional vegetables can contribute towards food diversity and food security, however, the benefits can only be reaped if the indigenous knowledge associated with traditional vegetables is available.

Chapter 6 - The literature has only recently begun to notice the cultural and emotional significance of familiar foods in supporting immigrants' healthy and deleterious eating practices in both their countries of origin and of destiny. The term *nostalgic foods* is used here to refer to the traditional food items and recipes prepared, eaten and maintained by immigrants and their families in the U.S., via everyday consumption and generational retention. While some aspects of traditional immigrants' diets may be protective against obesity and disease, particularly regarding the consumption of fruits and vegetables and the use of whole grains, some traditional eating patterns may be harmful, such as an excess of fried foods including chicken and plantains. This paper underscores the results of two focus group studies conducted with Latinas in New York City (NYC). The findings revealed that participants who experienced several hurdles in a new environment, tended to feel more "at home" via the preparation and consumption of culturally familiar foods. For many of them, traditional foods from their countries of origin (either raw items as mangoes or cooked items as plantains) provided "comfort," not just because of their taste and accessibility, but because they drew powerful emotional memories of the times spent either at their countries of origin or at family gatherings in the U.S. The study underscored paradoxical results regarding the selection of both healthy items (e.g., fruits and vegetables) and unhealthy items, such as staples heavily loaded with sugar (*buñuelos*, a kind of fried pastries) and fat (fried chicken). The authors' findings underscored interesting differences between first-generation immigrants (40 years and older) and younger second-generation Latinas (between 18 and 39 years old), regarding the meanings of "authentic" foods in their lives. While the first group preferred dishes that included the same ingredients and forms of preparation utilized in their countries of origin, second generation participants concocted their own notion of the "authentic," by introducing ingredients inspired by a wide sample of ethnic foods in NYC. The authors conclude this chapter by proposing a few possible health intervention strategies to be considered for promoting healthy eating among immigrant and minority groups. A better understanding of Latina's preferences, preparation and utilization of nostalgic foods will likely help inform future public health interventions towards improving, and preserving, Latinas' healthy eating habits and health.

Chapter 7 - Cucumber (*Cucumis sativus* L.) is cultivated widely as a vegetable crop. However, major parts of plants, such as stems, leaves and roots are mostly dumped as wastes at large expense after crop harvesting. Plants produce hundreds of secondary compounds and allelopathic active substances were found in cucumber plants. Allelopathic substance can provide a competitive advantage for host-plants through suppression of soil microorganism and inhibition of the growth of competing plant species because of their antibacterial, antifungal, and growth inhibitory activities. Allelopathy may represent a new frontier for the implementation of the practices applicable in the sustainable weed management strategies. In addition, allelopathic substances have potential as either herbicides or templates for new herbicide classes because of their strong herbicidal activity.

Chapter 8 - The characteristics of nitrogen nutrition and amino acid metabolism of cucumber plants were reviewed in relation to the nutritional values of fruits. The water content in cucumber fruits is high at about 95% based on the fresh weight. They contain organic compounds, such as sugars, proteins, vitamins, fibers and amino acids and inorganic minerals such as potassium. The major free amino acids in cucumber fruits were glutamine and citrulline, with alanine, serine and glycine at lower levels. The fruits of Gourd family (*Cucurbitaceae*) contain relatively large amount of citrulline, which is known to improve a human blood flow. In anthesis of female flower, citrulline was already present in the ovary, and its content increased with the growth of fruit. The most part of absorbed nitrogen (about 90%) was translocated from roots to the aerial parts though xylem vessels in the form of nitrate (NO_3^-). Thus the most part of NO_3^- was reduced to amino acids mainly in the leaves. However, a small part of the absorbed nitrogen was also reduced in the roots and subsequently translocated to the aerial parts as amino acids such as glutamine and citrulline. In leaves, citrulline accumulation occurred and it was the dominant free amino acids. Accumulation of ammonium in leaves was not observed possibly due to its toxicity. The absorbed nitrogen in the early stage of harvest was translocated rapidly to the leaves and assimilated there, then, the nitrogen in the leaves was retranslocated preferentially to the growing fruits. Based on ^{15}N analysis, approximately 50% of nitrogen contained in the harvested fruit was that absorbed after flowering of the fruit. Nitrogen absorbed before the harvest was also utilized in the formation of secondary lateral branches during fruit harevest period.

Chapter 9 - Since the United States Congress passed the Dietary Supplements and Health Education Act (DSHEA) in October of 1994, an herbal product can be classified as a nutritional supplement. For this reason, many of the products bought as nutritional supplements may contain herbs in some form or another. The DSHEA encouraged the marketing of diverse herbal products including teas, extracts, essential oils, syrups, used both for healing, as well as aesthetic purposes. The United States and Mexico share a very extensive international border, and studies suggest that herbal product use is even more common along the border area, compared to the rest of the country. Some people are still under the impression that because herbal products are “natural”, they are necessarily safe, and devoid of side effects. The lack of adequate quality control present in some herbal product companies around the world leads to variability in the quantity and quality of the products’ content. Serious intoxications have occurred around the globe due to mislabeling of herbal products or erroneous identification of some plant species. Interactions between herbal products and certain prescription and over the counter (OTC) medications can sometimes be serious. Various herbal supplements which are new to the U.S. market have not been adequately tested for purity, safety or efficacy. This chapter presents information regarding the safety of selected medicinal herbs used on the U. S. -Mexico border. Due to the lack of reliable clinical data regarding the safe use of various herbal products currently available, it is imperative that the public be aware about the possible health hazard of using certain herbs for therapeutic purposes.

Chapter 10 - *Background:* The importance and health benefits of vegetables are well known, while the nutritional requirements of older adults are different from those of younger adults. *Objective:* This study investigated vegetable consumption by gender and age groups among Japanese older adults. *Method:* A total of 558 eligible participants (341 men and 217 women) aged 55 to 75 years were recruited from 10 districts/prefectures in middle and southern Japan. Information on habitual vegetable consumption was obtained by face-to-face interviews using a validated and reliable food frequency questionnaire. *Results:* Women were found to consume more vegetables (mean 274, SD 166 g/day) than men (mean 207, SD 135 g/day) overall ($p < 0.001$) and across age groups 55-59, 60-64, 65-69 and 70-75 years. However, the intake levels of both genders did not vary significantly between age groups. The Japanese government has recommended an intake level of 350g or more per day for individuals. It is alarming that 83% of participants did not eat an adequate amount of vegetables. *Conclusion:* Japanese older adults especially men should be encouraged to increase their vegetable consumption in order to maintain their health and well-being.

In: Vegetable Consumption and Health: New Research
Editors: Claudia Wilson and Melinda Morree
ISBN: 978-1-62100-941-2

Chapter 1

FOOD INSECURITY AND VEGETABLE CONSUMPTION

Stephanie Grutzmacher, Susan Gross and Ashley Munger
Morgan State University, Center for Health Disparities Solutions, Public Health Program, Baltimore, Maryland, U. S.

ABSTRACT

Over 14.7% of U.S. households experienced food insecurity in 2009, while 21.3% of households with children under 18 and 22.9% of households with children under six were food insecure (Nord and Coleman-Jensen, 2010). In about 40% of food insecure households, one or more family members has experienced disruptions in normal eating patterns and reduced food intake due to limited resources. Low-income households are, unsurprisingly, less likely to purchase vegetables due to cost and availability and more likely to purchase affordable, energy-dense, nutrient-poor foods, which contain refined carbohydrates, added fats, and added sugars. Despite the availability of low-cost vegetable options in many communities, low-income mothers responsible for food purchasing and preparation perceive cost as a substantial barrier to vegetable consumption. Food insecurity may exacerbate some of the worrisome shopping and food consumption patterns observed in low-income households. One recent study of Latino households showed that household food insecurity was associated with lower quantities and less variety of fruits and vegetables in the home. Food insecurity is also related to decreased consumption of fruits and vegetables among adults as household resources deplete. Some studies have shown links between food insecurity and poor behavioral and academic outcomes for children, while other studies identified connections between parental psychological distress, family dysfunction, and low parent and child vegetable consumption. While few studies have attempted to parse out the causal pathway linking these various factors, it is possible that the stressful experiences and limited choices associated with poverty and food security undermine parents' abilities to access, afford, and provide healthful foods in the context of limited resources. Literature linking food insecurity with low vegetable consumption, however, is inconclusive, underscoring the need for improvements in study design to examine causal relationships between poverty, food insecurity, and vegetable consumption. In this chapter, we review the current state of knowledge on the indeterminate relationship between food security status and vegetable consumption, addressing the role of culture, the importance of safety net programs, and methodological issues.

INTRODUCTION

While most individuals do not consume the recommended amount of vegetables, vegetable expenditures and intake vary by household income [Bureau of Labor Statistics (BLS), 2010; Golan, Stewart, Kuchler, and Dong, 2008; Lorson Melgar-Quinonez, and Taylor, 2009; Munoz, Krebs-Smith, Ballard-Barbash, et al., 1997; Institute of Medicine (IOM), 2009]. Low-income individuals are less likely to buy fresh and processed vegetables than those with higher incomes (BLS, 2010). In 2009, the average annual household expenditure for fresh vegetables was $209, while the expenditure on fresh vegetables among the bottom-earning quintile was $126. Similarly, average expenditure for processed vegetables was $110, while the bottom quintile spent only $78 (BLS, 2010). Correspondingly, nutrient-dense foods like vegetables are costlier sources of dietary energy than refined grains, added sugars, and added fats (Drewnowski, 2010; Drewnowski and Darmon, 2005; Maillot, Darmon, and Drewnowski, 2010; Monsivais, Aggarwal, and Drewnowski, 2010; Monsivais and Drewnowski, 2009), further complicating low-income households' opportunities for consuming more vegetables. The cost of nutrient-dense foods is sharply increasing, while the cost of energy-dense foods is not (BLS, 2010; Monsivais and Drewnowski, 2007), underscoring the role of economic factors and agricultural policies in producing differential dietary quality outcomes in various socioeconomic groups. Limiting purchases of vegetables because of their high dietary energy cost may protect households struggling to afford needed quantities of food from greater food insecurity. As such, dietary quality is low among those with limited resources (Patterson, Haines, Popkin, 1994). These expenditure and consumption differences, in turn, may contribute to the widely observed health disparities in obesity and diet-related chronic diseases.

Low-income households are more likely to live in areas with limited access to fresh fruits and vegetables (Franco, Diez Roux, Glass, Caballero, and Brancati, 2008). Over four percent of the population is both low-income and living in a low-income area more than one mile from a supermarket [Economic Research Service (ERS), 2009]. In addition to access, cultural and social acceptability and other perceived barriers may further limit vegetable consumption among low-income households (Eikenberry and Smith, 2007; Glasson, Chapman, and James, 2011). Households must spend a larger portion of their time and money providing food (Golan, Stewart, Kuchler, and Dong, 2008).

While limited income itself is likely to function as a significant barrier to vegetable consumption, 43% of households living at or below the poverty line are also food insecure (Nord and Coleman-Jensen, 2011), possibly increasing risk for very low vegetable consumption. Food insecurity indicates limited resources for food spending and possible supplementation with emergency food resources such as those received from a food pantry. Particularly, food pantry clients report substituting canned and frozen vegetables for fresh vegetables (Hoisington, Schultz, and Butkus, 2002), signifying limited choice and variety available from emergency food services.

Despite some recent innovations like the addition of fruit and vegetable vouchers in the United States Department of Agriculture (USDA) programs including the Special Supplemental Program for Women, Infants, and Children (WIC) and the Fresh Fruit and Vegetable Program (FFVP), nutrition assistance programs have had limited success in substantially increasing the affordability or the perception of affordability of vegetables for low-income families.

Although it was not intended to cover all of a household's food expenses, the USDA's Supplemental Nutrition Assistance Program (SNAP) benefit allotments are predicated on an outdated assumption that households should spend about 30% of their income on food. SNAP covers all food costs in only one-third of households and in even fewer households in times of high food price inflation (Golan, Stewart, Kuchler, and Dong, 2008).

For example, the loss of purchasing power for a family of four grew from $12 at the beginning of the 2008 fiscal year to $56 in July before adjustments to benefit amounts based on the previous June's food prices occur (Golan, Stewart, Kuchler, and Dong, 2008). Food price inflation for food-at-home slowed between 2009 and 2010, resulting in a slight decline in vegetable prices after several years of high price inflation, but was projected to increase 3.5-4.5% in 2011 (Hanson and Andrews, 2008; Volpe and Leibtag, 2011).

Additionally, research showing a relationship between food stamp receipt and the purchase of larger amounts of fats and sugars (Wilde, McNamara, and Ranney, 2000) is one of the many reasons for a shift in the focus of SNAP from supplementing families' purchases to afford sufficient quantities of food to an increasing emphasis on dietary quality (Guthrie, Frazão, Andrews, and Smallwood, 2007).

Nevertheless, these changes are co-occurring with dramatic increases and record high SNAP enrollment and dramatic decreases in state and federal funding for SNAP benefits [Food and Nutrition Service (FNS), 2011].

The USDA's National School Lunch Program (NSLP), too, has the potential to improve children's vegetable access and fulfill a large portion of their dietary need for vegetables, but children often do not choose the vegetable meal components.

While these programs are an important resource for low-income families, they may not be achieving the goal of improving dietary quality.

Disparate Findings Regarding Food Security and Vegetable Consumption

Research has produced mixed results regarding the relationship between food insecurity and fruit and vegetable consumption. The findings of some studies indicate lower food security is related to lower fruit and vegetable consumption (Kendall, Olson, and Frongillo, 1996; Tingay, Tan, Tan, Tang, Teoh, Wong, and Gulliford, 2003; Tarasuk, McIntyre, and Li, 2007). Kendall, Olson, and Frongillo (1996) investigated a random sample of 193 women in rural New York. In-home interviews were conducted and included the Radimer/Cornell hunger and food insecurity scale, questions regarding the frequency of fruit and vegetable consumption from the Centers for Disease Control and Prevention's (CDC) Behavioral Risk Factor Surveillance System (BRFSS), 24-hour dietary recall, and a household food inventory conducted by the researchers in the homes of the participants. In the sample, 46.6% were classified as food secure, while 53.4% were classified as food insecure. Lower food security was significantly associated with less frequent consumption of fruits and vegetables and a lower percentage of participants consuming the recommended daily allowance of fruit and vegetables; however, neither the food secure group nor the food insecure group consumed the recommended daily servings of fruits and vegetables.

In a national study using the National Health and Nutrition Examination Survey (NHANES)-III data, 6,475 White, Black, or Mexican American adults from food insufficient families were more likely to report less frequent consumption of fruit/fruit juices and vegetables than adults from food secure families (Dixon, 2001). Tingay and colleagues (2003) studied food insecurity in inner London. The 431 participants completed the short form Household Food Security Survey Module (HFSSM) and a short food frequency questionnaire from the Health Survey for England 1994. Of the participants, 20% were classified as food insecure. Food security in the sample was negatively associated with household income and level of education. Those who were food insecure were significantly less likely to report daily fruit and vegetable consumption.

Olson (2005) found that women may be particularly at risk. Women's roles in managing family feeding made them more vulnerable to food insecurity; women sacrificed fruit and vegetable intake as periods of hunger approached. The reduced intakes of fruits and vegetables among food insecure women resulted in significantly lower nutrient intakes (Olson, 2005). In addition, Tarasuk, McIntyre, and Li (2007) studied 180 low-income Canadian women who receive most of their income from one check per month to determine how dwindling resources during the month coincided with their food consumption. Data were combined from two studies that used periodic 24-hour dietary recalls to assess food consumption. One of the studies used the HFSSM to assess food security status, while the other used the Radimer/Cornell instrument. Equivalency was established between the adult measures of food security on these two instruments. Most of the women were White, had children and received their main source of income from social assistance. Sixty-five percent of the sample was moderately to severely food insecure. Combined fruit and vegetable intake and vegetable intake alone (excluding potatoes) were significantly related to the number of days since the receipt of income for those who reported moderate or severe food insecurity, but not for those who reported food security or marginal food security. Findings from these studies emphasize the role of mothers in protecting children from food insecurity and hunger and the temporal and fluctuating nature of the food insecure experience.

In one cross-sectional study of 928 frequent food pantry users, food security and self-reported health information were collected in face-to-face interviews at 58 different pantry locations in central and northeast Missouri. Each one-point increase on the food security scale (indicating greater food insecurity) resulted in a .564 decrease in all fruit and vegetable intake (Raedeke, 2007). In another study of children of recent Somali refugee migrant workers (n=35), 72% of the families were food insecure, and consumption of green leafy vegetables was lower in food insecure households (Dharod, 2011). A third study of postpartum WIC participants (n=155) showed strong links between food security and vegetable consumption. Food insecure participants were 8.8 times as likely to report low vegetable consumption (seldom/never eating 2.5 cups of vegetables per day) than food secure participants, after adjusting for age, income, education, and ethnicity (Mathews, Morris, Schneider, and Goto, 2010).

Other studies, however, have found no such relationship. For instance, Dave and colleagues (2009) studied food insecurity and children's fruit and vegetable consumption in a convenience sample of 184 parents of Hispanic children aged 5 to 12. Food insecurity was assessed using two food security items on the Food Behavior Checklist, while fruit and vegetable consumption was assessed using the short Block screener form. Results indicated that total fruit and vegetable consumption did not vary significantly between food secure and food insecure groups. However, parents of children in food secure households reported that children consume more fresh and canned fruit and more vegetable juice than children in food insecure households, indicating that measuring fruits and vegetables, juices, and canned, frozen, and fresh forms separately may improve understanding of vegetable consumption patterns among food secure and food insecure households.

Surprisingly, others have found that lower food security is associated with increased fruit and/or vegetable consumption (Lorson, Melgar-Quinonez, and Taylor, 2009; Stuff et al., 2009; Mello, Gans, Risica, Kirtania, Strolla, and Fournier, 2010). Lorson and colleagues (2009) investigated the correlates of fruit and vegetable consumption among 6,513 children and adolescents (ages 2 - 18) surveyed during the 1999 - 2002 waves of NHANES. Household income was significantly associated with total fruit intake (measured using 24-hour dietary recalls), with households with incomes between 130% and 350% of the federal poverty line consuming less fruit than households with higher incomes. However, there were no significant differences by income level for total vegetable intake. The differences in fruit and vegetable consumption across food security statuses were not significant, though a trend for those with lower food security to consume more fruit than those with higher food security was observed. However, this finding was explained by higher fruit juice consumption among food insecure households. The researchers also found that Mexican American children and adolescents were two-thirds more likely to consume fruit than their non-Hispanic White counterparts. Most of the sample did not meet the fruit or vegetable intake recommendations, regardless of food security status or income.

In a study of multiethnic middle and high school students, food security was measured by hunger frequency and home food adequacy as reported by the students. Over eight percent of students reported hunger. Students who were food insecure appeared to be more likely to meet Healthy People 2010 goals related to vegetable intake than were their food secure peers, but the number of adolescents meeting these targets was low for all groups. Students reporting hunger may have had greater access to vegetables through nutrition assistance programs such as NSLP, food pantries, afterschool programs, or meals served at shelters (Widome, Neumark-Sztainer, Hannan, Haines, and Story, 2009).

In another study, Stuff and colleagues (2009) assessed food security, as measured by the 6-item HFSSM, and dietary intake, as measured by two partial and one full 24-hour recalls, in a multiethnic sample of 688 parents of children in Texas and Alabama Head Start programs. Prevalence of food insecurity in the sample was 34.9%. Food insecure children consumed more servings of fruit and vegetables than food secure children; however, neither group consumed the recommended daily servings. The researchers note that Latina mothers in other studies consumed more servings of fruits and vegetables than their non-Latina counterparts, despite their high risk for food insecurity. Although not explicitly identified by Stuff and colleagues as an explanation for their findings, juice consumption may account for higher levels of fruit and vegetable consumption among food insecure children.

Mello and colleagues (2010) examined the relationship between food insecurity and dietary behaviors in a sample of 1,874 multiethnic, low-income adults. Food security status, as measured by the food security question from the BRFSS, was not significantly associated with fruit and vegetable consumption, as measured by the Fruit and Vegetable Frequency Questionnaire. When fruit juice consumption was included in fruit intakes, food insecure individuals consumed more fruit than those who were food secure; however, when adjusted for demographic characteristics, no differences were observed. The authors postulate that their adjustment for demographic variables may explain why they did not find the association between food security and fruit and vegetable consumption found in other analyses that did not control for demographic characteristics.

Low Fruit and Vegetable Consumption

Among the reviewed studies, many of the samples had a low prevalence of adequate fruit and vegetable consumption (Kendall, Olson, and Frongillo, 1996; Kilanowski and Moore, 2010; Lorson, Melgar-Quinonez, and Taylor, 2009; Stuff et al., 2009). These studies primarily investigated low-income individuals. Kamphuis and colleagues (2006) examined the association between fruit and vegetable consumption, socioeconomic status, and perceptions regarding food availability, accessibility, and affordability in a sample of Australian women and determined that these perceptions mediated the relationship between fruit and vegetable consumption and education, but not income. It is possible that people of similar income levels develop similar perceptions regarding fruit and vegetable accessibility and affordability, which may pose a barrier to the purchase of fruits and vegetables.

However, not only low-income individuals consume less than the recommended amounts of fruits and vegetables. Low fruit and vegetable consumption reflects a national trend. Research has shown that, in general, individuals in the United States do not consume the recommended amounts of fruits and vegetables, even though fruit and vegetable intake has been strongly linked to myriad positive health outcomes (Nöthlings, Schulze, Weichart, et al., 2008). According to the CDC, in 2009, no state met the Healthy People 2010 goals regarding fruit and vegetable consumption. The stated aim was to increase the proportion of those two years of age and older who consume two or more daily servings of fruit to 75% and to increase the proportion of those who consume three or more daily servings of vegetables to 50%. According to the 2009 BRFSS, approximately 32.5% of U.S. adults consumed two or more servings of fruit per day and 26.3% consumed three or more servings of vegetables per day. Latinos consumed the most fruit and the fewest vegetables, perhaps reflecting distinctive cultural food preferences. The proportions of those eating two or more servings of fruit among various income levels were comparable, with 32.2%, 31.4%, 32.9%, and 32% of those earning less than $25,000, those earning between $25,000 and $49,999, those earning more than $50,000, and those with unknown income, respectively. The proportions of those consuming three or more servings of vegetables per day were 22.0%, 24.8%, 29.4%, and 21.8% of those earning less than $25,000, those earning between $25,000 and $49,999, those earning more than $50,000, and those with unknown income, respectively. With such limited variability in fruit and vegetable consumption, it is possible that differences would be hard to detect, particularly in the small samples found in many of the studies investigating fruit and vegetable consumption in the context of food insecurity. Moreover, research examining relationships between income and fruit and vegetable consumption (Inglis, Ball, and Crawford, 2007; Kamphuis et al., 2006) produce inconsistent results similar to the literature addressing food security and fruit and vegetable consumption. These inconsistencies may largely be attributable to methodological issues such as sampling, control variables, and selection effects.

Cultural Factors

The disparate findings regarding the relationship between food security and fruit and vegetable consumption may also reflect cultural factors, such as acculturation and cultural fruit and vegetable preferences.

This may be especially true in studies that found an association between lower food security and increased fruit and vegetable consumption, as Latinos experience disproportionately low levels of food security (USDA, 2011) but also evince greater levels of fruit and vegetable consumption with lower levels of acculturation. Dave and colleagues (2009) found that Latino children who were more acculturated to the US, based on home language preference, consumed fewer fruits and vegetables than children in less acculturated families. In this sample, fruit and vegetable consumption was not significantly different between the food secure and food insecure groups. The researchers stated that, "this finding suggests that the traditional Latino diet, which less-acculturated individuals tend to eat, forms a culture-based protection, or buffering, against poor dietary patterns" (Dave et al., 2009, p.699).

Similarly, Neuhouser and colleagues (2004) found that greater acculturation among Hispanic immigrants from Mexico was associated with lower fruit and vegetable intakes. Acculturation among Somali refugees in the US was associated with increased intake of snack food items (Dharod, Croom, Sady, and Morrell, 2011). Adoption of more mainstream American dietary practices may account for observed declines in vegetable consumption as immigrants live in the United States longer. These findings provide support for a health behavior and acculturation hypothesis to explain the Latino mortality paradox, which refers to Latino's overall better health despite lower socioeconomic status (Abraido-Lanza, Chao, and Florez, 2005; Lara, Gambo, Kahramanian, Morales, and Bautista, 2005).

In addition to ethnicity, other cultural factors related to preferences and access may play a role in explaining the relationship between food security and vegetable consumption. In one study of rural and urban low-income caretakers, vegetable intake and variety of vegetables were greater for rural families compared with urban families (Haldeman, Gruber, and Ingram, 2008). Store type, quality, and cost available in communities may also influence shopping decisions, and thus vegetable purchases, for low-income families. In one study, participants who shopped at Big Box stores with an operation offering more than food (such as Wal-Mart) purchased fewer vegetables than participants who shopped at grocery stores (Dammann, Smith, and Race, 2010).

Similar results related to store type, store environment, and other store qualities were reported by Zenk and colleagues (2005) and Webber and colleagues (2010). In a study of a low-income neighborhood stores, less than 50% of the stores carried commonly consumed and culturally specific vegetables preferred by Latino and African American residents (Grigsby-Toussant, Zenk, Odoms-Young, Ruggiero, and Moise, 2010). Because access to vegetables is cited as a barrier to vegetable consumption for low-income households, perhaps the even more limited availability of culturally-specific vegetables further undermines ethnic minority families' vegetable purchasing.

Impact of Safety Nets

The ambiguous findings regarding food security and vegetable consumption may also reflect the impact of food safety nets, which provide additional food resources, such as produce vouchers and nutrition education classes, to low-income individuals. Food assistance programs in the United States such as WIC and SNAP seek to alleviate food insecurity-related dietary problems. Yet, it is challenging to design studies that adequately control for selection effects of program participation. Many eligible individuals do not enroll in available programs for various reasons, including stigma, difficulty with paperwork, and access to other protective resources. Other low-income individuals may fluctuate between eligible and ineligible, while those whose incomes linger just above eligibility may be as at-risk for food insecurity as those who are eligible, but they will not be able to participate in protective nutrition assistance programs.

In an evaluation of a Maryland nutrition education program focusing on fruit and vegetable consumption, Havas and colleagues (1998) found that, compared with controls, those in the class increased fruit and vegetable consumption by an average one-half serving daily. The number of nutrition education classes attended, ethnicity, education, and self-efficacy were all significant predictors of fruit and vegetable consumption. Kropf (2007) found that more food insecure participants in an intervention group receiving WIC Farmers' Market Voucher perceived diet quality to be "very good or excellent" compared with food insecure participants in the control group (30.8% vs. 15.9%). In addition, Herman, Harrison, Afifi, and Jenks (2008) studied 608 Los Angeles women participating in WIC who were assigned to receive either farmers' market fruit and vegetable vouchers, supermarket fruit and vegetable vouchers, or a non-food incentive during a six-month intervention period. The sample was 89.1% Latino, and 39.4% of the women were food insecure. Farmers' market and supermarket intervention participants increased fruit and vegetable consumption compared with those in the control group. Changes were sustained at the six-month follow-up. The differences were significant, even when excluding beans, potatoes, and juices from fruit and vegetable intake. Higher fruit and vegetable consumption at the six-month follow-up was associated with higher baseline fruit and vegetable consumption and a preference for speaking Spanish[1]. Tarasuk, McIntyre, and Li's (2007) study also indicates the importance of food assistance for those who are moderately to severely food insecure, as fruit and vegetable consumption decreased when monetary resources in the house dwindled. Researchers whose samples consist of those who are low-income may find that those with the lowest incomes

[1] It should be noted that the studies discussed in this chapter examine vegetable intakes of WIC participants receiving the old WIC food package, which only included juice and fresh carrots to breastfeeding women. These items may highlight the role of juice in increasing overall fruit and vegetable intake in studies that did not measure juice separately and explain some of the inconsistencies in the relationship between fruit and vegetable consumption and food security. Additionally, future studies of WIC participants' may reflect higher vegetable intakes.

who are food insecure have developed effective coping strategies to attain fruits and vegetables through the aid of public safety nets.

WIC and SNAP are widely explored as protective of food insecurity, but other nutrition assistance programs such as Child and Adult Care Food Program (CACFP) and NSLP also play a role in the food security status of adults and children and may impact overall vegetable consumption. In a study of low-income elementary students and their parents, students from low food security households who were also not participating in the school nutrition programs had the lowest vegetable consumption in the sample (Grutzmacher and Gross, 2011). Additionally, these students consumed breakfast on the fewest number of days. While most students and parents in the study had low vegetable intake, the students in food insecure households who were not enrolled in school meals may have had a greater need for enrollment than their peers from food secure households. This study illustrates the importance of increasing enrollment in school nutrition programs and considering these programs as a vehicle for increasing children's vegetable consumption.

Some nutrition assistance programs like SNAP or purchase incentive programs aim to lower the cost of food purchases. Yet, perceptions of food availability and cost often drive vegetable consumption behavior (Bihan, Castetbon, and Mejean, 2010, Dibsdall, Lambert, Bobbin, and Frewer, 2003; Inglis, Ball, and Crawford, 2008). In one study, the associations between socio-economic status and diet were weak and non-significant, suggesting that socioeconomic differences in diet were almost wholly explained by perceptions of food availability, accessibility and affordability (Inglis, Ball and Crawford, 2008). Among low-income adults, perceptions of lack of affordability of fruits and vegetables were related to low consumption of vegetables (Giskes, van Lenthe, Kamphuis, et al., 2009; Havas, Treiman, and Langenberg, 1998). A study of low-income adults reported that the majority of respondents perceived healthy foods as costlier, but also indicated that they would be willing to purchase healthy foods if they cost less (Peterson, Dodd, Kim, and Roth, 2010). Future research should address whether perceptions match objective measures of food availability, accessibility and affordability in order to address the real and/or perceived lack of healthy options in low-income neighborhoods.

Overall, findings regarding the relationship between vegetable consumption and food security are inconclusive, largely due to methodological issues like food security measurement, sampling, vegetable intake measurement, confounding variables, program enrollment selection effects, and cross-sectional observations. These issues and recommendations for future research will be discussed.

Conceptualizing and Measuring Food Security

Definition and Classification

While food insecurity has long been a concern in the United States, the recent economic downturn, shrinking public and private safety nets, and poor health outcomes associated with poverty have heightened worry over the rise in food insecurity prevalence. In 2009, 14.7% of US households experienced food insecurity, the highest recorded prevalence since data collection began in 1995 (Nord, Coleman-Jensen, Andrews, and Carlson, 2010). *Food insecurity,* the limited or uncertain availability of nutritionally adequate and safe foods or limited or uncertain ability to acquire acceptable foods in socially acceptable ways (Anderson, 1990. pp. 1575-1576), is associated with a wide variety of negative outcomes for adults (American Dietetic Association, 2010; Stuff, Casey, Szeto, et al., 2004) and children (Matheson, Varady, and Varady, 2002; Smith and Richards, 2008). The USDA defines food security as access by all people at all times to enough food for an active, healthy life. Food security includes (1) the ready availability of nutritionally adequate and safe foods and (2) an assured ability to acquire acceptable foods in socially acceptable ways (e.g., without resorting to emergency food supplies, scavenging, stealing, or other coping strategies) (Anderson, 1990).

In 2005, the USDA changed the food security classifications for the FSS and HFSSM from food secure, food insecure without hunger, food insecure with hunger and food insecure with child hunger (Bickel, Nord, Price, Hamilton, and Cook, 2000) to the following: High food security (households show no or minimal evidence of food insecurity); Marginal food security (food insecurity is evident in household members' concerns about adequacy of the household food supply and in adjustments to household food management, including reduced quality of food and increased unusual coping patterns. Little or no reduction in members' food intake is reported); Low food security (food intake for adults in the household has been reduced to an extent that implies that adults have repeatedly experienced the physical sensation of hunger. In most, but not all, food insecure households with children, such reductions are not observed at this stage for children); and Very low food security (all households with children have reduced the children's food intake to an extent indicating that the children have experienced hunger. For some other households with children, this already has occurred at an earlier stage of severity. Adults in households with and without children have repeatedly experienced more extensive reductions in food intake). The wording of the questionnaire remained unchanged. Although the word *hungry* was retained in the questions (Nord, Coleman-Jensen, Andrews, and Carlson, 2010), *hunger* was eliminated from the new classifications. The USDA removed hunger from definitions because the physiologic experience of hunger was not adequately assessed in the food security questions (Nord, Coleman-Jensen, Andrews, and Carlson, 2010). It is noted that low food security and very low food security continue to be collectively referred to as food insecure (Nord, Coleman-Jensen, Andrews, and Carlson, 2010).

Measurement

Since 1995, the rate of food insecurity in the United States has been tracked and measured by the USDA using the HFSSM (American Dietetic Association, 2010; Nord, Coleman-Jensen, Andrews, and Carlson, 2010). Data is collected by survey once a year as a supplement to the Current Population Survey, conducted by the U.S. Census Bureau (Nord, Coleman-Jensen, Andrews, and Carlson, 2010). The number of questions is dependent upon whether children are present in the home. The module is comprised of 18 questions for households with children and 10 questions for households without children. While the HFSSM does not measure food intake, it does examine factors influencing food intake. The HFSSM questions address the following: fear and anxiety related to the insufficiency of the food budget to meet basic needs; food shortages without having the financial resources to purchase more; perceived quality and quantity of food consumed by household members;

atypical food usage, such as substituting fewer or cheaper foods; and episodes of reduced food intake, hunger or weight loss by household members (Bickel, Nord, Price, Hamilton, and Cook, 2000; Blumberg, Bialostosky, Briefel, and Hamilton, 1999). The questions are intended to measure whether a household is food secure and the severity of food insecurity. Each question references a specific timeframe, either the past 12 months or the past 30 days.

A shorter, six-question format, the Food Security Supplement (FSS) has also been used to more rapidly assess household food security (Bickel, Nord, Price, Hamilton, and Cook, 2000). This standard short form has shown reasonably high specificity and sensitivity and minimal bias with respect to the 18-question measure (Blumberg, Bialostosky, Briefel, and Hamilton, 1999). A limitation of using the shortened scale, however, is the inability to identify households with child hunger, as the measure only assesses household food insecurity (Bickel, Nord, Price, Hamilton, and Cook, 2000). Because of its brevity, this measure is commonly used by researchers.

Measurement of child food insecurity also proves to be problematic. The 18 items in the HFSSM measures two dimensions of food security, adult food insecurity and child food insecurity. These two dimensions are correlated but not collinear (Nord and Bickel, 2002; Nord and Hopwood, 2007). The correlation depends on the ages of children (Nord and Hopwood, 2007). As a result, underestimation of food security for adults can occur. To address this problem, Nord and Bickel (2002) developed the Children's Food Security Scale, which includes only the eight child-referenced items in the standard module. The Child Food Security Survey Module was developed by adapting questions from the HFSSM for direct administration to children ages 6-12 and 12-15. Separate measures of children's and adults' food security appear to provide better assessment than a single measure that attempts to represent both (Nord and Hopwood, 2007). This scale has been validated in low-income populations (Nord and Hopwood, 2007).

The Radimer/Cornell food insecurity measure is another commonly used food security measure. It is based on the conceptual framework that food insecurity is experienced differently at the household level and at the individual level, and the experience differs between adults and children at the individual level. The components of the framework at each level (household, adult, and child) contain the food available to the household or consumed by individuals and the psychological and social components experienced by households and individuals. Food insecurity is conceptualized as a continuum that progresses from uncertainty and anxiety about food at the household level to the extreme condition of hunger among children when they do not have enough to eat. Studies in the United States have reported strong criterion validity (Kendall, Olson, and Frongillo, 1995) and good internal consistency. In addition, this scale has been validated in many other countries around the world (Derrikson, Fisher, and Anderson, 2000; Frongillo, Raushenbach, Olson, et al., 1997). In relation to criterion-related validity examined in one study, as food insecurity worsened, there was a significant and progressive increase in the percentage of subjects participating in food programs and having low income, education and employment, as well as a significant decline in average household food availability and fruit and vegetable consumption (Kendall, Olson, and Frongillo, 1995). Components of the HFSSM were adapted from this scale. This scale yields detail about the household, adult, and child experiences of food insecurity, which may help researchers more accurately assess the variable and nested nature of food insecurity within households.

Another common measure of food insecurity uses the two food security items on the Food Behavior Checklist, which were utilized to enable nutrition educators to assess the level of economic constraints among participants. Townsend and colleagues (2003) validated the two-item index on a four-point response scale for measuring food security with a low-income population. Responses to the two food insecurity items were highly correlated ($r = .85$). The item “Do you run out of food before the end of the month?” was correlated with both the percent of energy from fat and fruit intake (Townsend, Kaiser, and Allen, 2003). Based on this finding, the authors concluded that their measures met criterion validity standards since other studies had also demonstrated that food insecurity is significantly correlated with lower household stores of fruit and vegetables and with increased calories from fat. This measure, while not appropriate for detailed information about household food insecurity, may help identify those at risk for food insecurity in community-based nutrition education settings in which time for needs assessment and evaluation is quite limited.

Project EAT (Widome, Neumark-Sztainer, Hannan, Haines, and Story, 2009) adapted two items from the Food Security/Hunger Core Module (ERS, 1999). The first item, which measured "hunger frequency,"was "How often during the last 12 months have you been hungry because your family couldn't afford food?" The response categories were (1) almost every month, (2) some months but not every month, (3) only 1 or 2 months, and (4) I have not been hungry for this reason. The second item, which measured "home food adequacy," was "Which of these statements best describes the food eaten in your home in the last 12 months?" The response categories were (1) often we don't have enough to eat, (2) sometimes we don't have enough to eat, (3) we have enough to eat but not always the kinds of foods we want, and (4) we always have enough to eat and the kinds of foods we want.

The strength of Project EAT’s food security measurement was that it targeted the adolescents’ food security levels. This is an improvement over questions asked of household adults, because food security issues may affect various members in a household to differing extents (Nord, Andrews, and Carlson, 2007). However, the Project EAT food security questions were not extensively validated. These items attempt to assess frequency of hunger and adequacy of variety/choice and quantity, which may function as a rapid food security screener.

Further examination of the role of culture in perceptions and experiences of food insecurity is needed to ensure that food insecurity measures are appropriate and valid across cultural contexts. In an analysis of food insecurity studies across multiple cultures, Coates and colleagues (2006) identified common themes in food security from several cultures. Their analysis confirmed that insufficient food quantity, inadequate food quality, and uncertainty and worry about food were significant parts of the food insecurity experience in all sampled cultures. Concerns about social unacceptability emerged in all ethnographic accounts (Coates, Frongillo, and Lorge Rogers, 2006). The HFSSM does not fully represent all potentially important domains and sub domains of the food insecurity experience.

Methodological Challenges in Examining Food Security-Dietary Quality Relationships

The experience of food security is cyclic in nature, with households vacillating between food availability after receiving SNAP benefits or paychecks and food insufficiency, meal skipping, and other disruptions in normal eating patterns (Cook, Frank, Berkowitz, et al., 2004; Guilliford, Nunes, and Rocke, 2006; Kaiser, Melgar- Quiñonez, Lamp, Sutherlin, Johns, and Harwood, 2002; Townsend, Peerson, Love, Achterberg, and Murphy, 2001; Wilde and Ranney, 1998; Wilde and Peterman, 2006). The reference period used in food security assessment can also alter the meaning of observed relationships with dietary behaviors. Using the HFSSM, food insecurity is typically indicated by an experience of measured conditions *any time* during the previous 12 months, whereas the reference period for vegetable consumption is typically the previous 24 hours or seven days. For example, a household experiencing a single episode of hunger may be classified as food insecure, but recent vegetable consumption in the household reflects behavior under more normal circumstances for the household. Researchers would need to interpret any observed relationships (or lack of observed relationships) between food security over the previous 12 months and vegetable consumption on the previous day cautiously because it may not be possible to determine whether food insecurity is a rare or chronic state. The Economic Research Service examined how often people in food insecure with hunger households were hungry. Findings indicated that approximately one-third of households that were food insecure with hunger at any time during the year experienced the condition rarely or occasionally, and that approximately 30% of food insecure with hunger households had frequent or chronic occurrence, meaning that hunger occurred almost every month (Nord, Coleman-Jensen, Andrews, and Carlson, 2010). Clearly, households experiencing chronic hunger could report markedly different dietary patterns and behaviors than households rarely experiencing hunger.

Food insecurity differentially affects adults and children, men and women, individuals with and without instrumental social support, and individuals who are enrolled, eligible but not enrolled, and non-eligible for nutrition assistance programs. Community dimensions like food availability and accessibility (generally and culturally specific) and cost and economic dimensions like food price inflation and nutrition assistance benefit levels also impact the experience of food insecurity for various households differently. Thus, measurement of frequency, severity, and nature of food insecurity experiences is quite challenging. Longitudinal data may help elucidate temporal patterns in the food insecurity experiences of low-income households.

Challenges with the measurement of vegetable consumption may be addressed elsewhere in this volume. Studies addressing vegetable consumption among low-income or food insecure households indicate a strong need to measure fruit, fruit juice, vegetable, and vegetable juice consumption separately (e.g., Glasson, Chapman, and James, 2011). There may be additional utility to isolating quantities of energy-dense or starchy vegetables in assessing vegetable intake. Taste preferences, nutrient density, affordability, and other factors indicate different consumption patterns for fruits, vegetables, and juices, therefore the large number of studies aggregating fruit, vegetable, and juice consumption into one construct may obscure patterns and associations with important implications for social marketing, nutrition education, and policy interventions. Additionally, many studies measure vegetable intake in one setting (e.g., schools or homes), decreasing accuracy and utility.

Many studies addressing food insecurity and dietary outcomes utilize non-representative samples of individuals recruited through Supplemental Nutrition Assistance Program Nutrition Education (SNAP-Ed), Expanded Food and Nutrition Education Program (EFNEP), WIC, or other programs. Samples recruited via these programs may introduce significant selection bias due to their eligibility, enrollment, and participation. Furthermore, data collection in such settings, particularly those conducted as a part of program evaluations, tend to require rapid assessment of several complex phenomena. At a minimum, researchers should collect data on and address confounding variables such as education, program participation, and income.

CONCLUSION

Overall, few studies examine the relationship between food security and vegetable consumption systematically with representative samples, longitudinal data, and congruent reference periods. Most studies combine fruit and vegetable consumption, despite evidence that consumption and barriers to consumption differ between these two food categories (Glasson, Chapman, and James, 2011). More knowledge is needed to understand the patterns of food insecurity and vegetable consumption, as neither of these phenomena are static or consistent behaviors. The role of nutrition assistance programs as indicators of risk (e.g., the need to enroll) and resources (e.g., the receipt of helpful benefits) also merits continued examination. Additional qualitative research to examine the food insecurity experiences and individuals' perceptions may also help identify constructs and confounders that should be included in assessments of food security.

While few studies have attempted to parse out the causal pathway linking food insecurity with various negative outcomes, it is possible that the stressful experiences and limited choices associated with poverty and food security undermine individuals' abilities to access, afford, and provide healthful foods in the context of limited resources. Literature linking food insecurity with low vegetable consumption, however, is inconclusive, underscoring the need for improvements in study design to examine causal relationships between poverty, food insecurity, and vegetable consumption.

Despite anxiety about affording enough food itself being problematic, food insecure households not experiencing overt hunger can attend to qualitative or nutritional aspects of the diet more so than the most vulnerable households, for which the concern of having enough food overrides the concerns about food quality (Coates, Frongillo, and Lorge Rogers, 2006). Many adults in households with low food security alter their food intake when resources deplete (Tarasuk, McIntyre, and Li, 2007). It is important to consider that while children may be protected from meal skipping and other disruptions to dietary patterns, parents' disruptive experiences may negatively influence their child feeding behaviors and other aspects of the home nutrition environment that indeed affect children. Examination of such characteristics over time may expose connections between adult and household food insecurity and adult and child dietary outcomes.

REFERENCES

Abraido-Lanza AF, Chao MT, Florez KR. Do healthy behaviors decline with greater acculturation? Implications for the Latino mortality paradox. *Soc Sciences and Med., September* 2005;61(6):1243-1255.

American Dietetic Association. Position of the American Dietetic Association: Food insecurity in the United States. *J. Am. Diet Assoc.,* September 2010;110(9):1368-77.

Anderson S. Core indicators of nutritional state for difficult to sample populations. *J. Nutr.* 1990;102:1559-1660.

Bickel G, Nord M, Price C, Hamilton W, Cook J. *Guide to Measuring Household Food Security,* Revised 2000. U.S. Department of Agriculture, Food and Nutrition Service, Alexandria, VA: March 2000:1-82.

Bihan H, Castetbon K, Mejean C, et al. Sociodemographic factors and attitudes toward food affordability and health are associated with fruit and vegetable consumption in a low-income French population. *J. Nutr.*, 2010;140: 823-30.

Blumberg SJ, Bialostosky K, Briefel RR, Hamilton WL. The effectiveness of a short form of the household food security scale. *Am. J. Public Health.*, 1999;89:1231-1234.

Bureau of Labor Statistics. 2009 Consumer Expenditure Survey Data. Washington, D.C.: U.S. Department of Labor, Bureau of Labor Statistics, 2010. Accessed August 4, 2011.

Centers for Disease Control and Prevention. State-specific trends in fruit and vegetable consumption among adults-United States, 2000-2009. *Morbidity and Mortality Weekly Report.* September 10 2010;59(35);1125-*1130.* http://www.cdc.gov/mmwr/preview/mmwrhtml/mm5935a1.htm. Accessed July 10, 2011.

Coates J, Frongillo EA, Lorge Rogers B, et al. Commonalities in the experience of household food insecurity across cultures: What are measures missing? *J. Nutr.,* 2006;136:1438S-1448S.

Cook JT, Frank DF, Berkowitz C, et al. Food insecurity is associated with adverse health outcomes among human infants and toddlers. *J. Nutr.*, 2004;134:1432-1438.

Dammann KW, Smith C. Race, homelessness, and other environmental factors associated with the food-purchasing behavior of low-income women. *J. Am. Diet Assoc.*, 2010;110:1351-1356.

Dave JM, Evans AE, Pfeiffer KA, Watkins KW, Saunders RP. Correlates of availability and accessibility of fruits and vegetables in homes of low-income Hispanic families. *Health Educ. Res.*, 2010;25(1):97-108.

Dave JM, Evans AE, Saunders RP, Watkins KW, Pfeiffer KA. Associations among food insecurity, acculturation, demographic factors, and fruit and vegetable intake at home in Hispanic children. *J. Am. Diet Assoc.*, 2009;109(4):697-701.

Dehghan M, Akhtar-Danesh N, Merchant AT. Factors associated with fruit and vegetable consumption among adults. *J. Hum. Nutr. Diet.* 2011;24(2):128-134.

Derrickson JP, Fisher AG, Anderson JE. The core food security module scale measure is valid and reliable when used with Asians and Pacific Islanders. *J. Nutr.*. November 2000;130(11):2666-2674.

Dharod JM, Croom J, Sady CG, Morrell D. Dietary intake, food security, and acculturation among Somali refugees in the United States: Results of a pilot study. *J. Immigr. Refug. Stud.*, 2011;9(1):82–97.

Dibsdall LA, Lambert N, Bobbin RF, Frewer LJ. Low-income consumers' attitudes and behaviour towards access, availability and motivation to eat fruit and vegetables. *Public Health Nutr.*, April 2003;6(2):159-68.

Dixon LB, Winkleby MA, Radimer KL. Dietary intakes and serum nutrients differ between adults from food-insufficient and food-sufficient families: Third National Health and Nutrition Examination Survey, 1988-1994. *J. Nutr.*, 2001;131:1232-1246.

Dong D, Lin B. Fruit and vegetable consumption by low-income Americans: Would a price reduction make a difference? *Economic research report*, January 2009;70:1-17.

Drewnowski A. The cost of US foods as related to their nutritive value. *Am J Clin. Nutr.* November 2010;92(5):1181-1188.

Drewnowski A, Darmon N. The economics of obesity: Dietary energy density and energy cost. *Am. J. Clin. Nutr.,* 2005;82:265S-273S.

Economic Research Service. Access to Affordable and Nutritious Food: Measuring and Understanding Food Deserts and Their Consequences. Administrative Publication AP-036. Washington, DC: US Department of Agriculture; 2009. http://www.ers.usda.gov/ Publications/AP/AP036/ AP036.pdf. Accessed August 2, 2011.

Economic Research Service. Food Security/Hunger Core Module: 3-Stage Design, With Screeners. Washington, DC: US Department of Agriculture, Food and Nutrition Service and Economic Research Service; 1999. http://www.ers.usda.gov/briefing/foodsecurity/ surveytools/core0699.pdf. Accessed June 29, 2011.

Eikenberry N, Smith C. Healthful eating: Perceptions, motivations, barriers, and promoters in low-income Minnesota communities. *J. Am. Diet. Assoc.,* 2007;104(7):1158-1161.

Food and Nutrition Service. FNS Program Data – SNAP. Food and Nutrition Service, United States Department of Agriculture. http://www.fns.usda.gov/ pd/snapmain.htm. Accessed August 7, 2011.

Frongillo EA, Raushenbach BS, Olson CM, Kendall A and Colmenares AG. Questionnaire-based measures are valid for the identification of rural households with hunger and food insecurity. *J. Nutr.*, 1997;127:699-705.

Giskes K, van Lenthe FJ, Kamphuis CB, Huisman M, Brug J, Mackenbach JP. Household and food shopping environments: Do they play a role in socioeconomic inequalities in fruit and vegetable consumption? A multilevel study among Dutch adults. *J. Epidemiol. Community Health.,* 2009;63:113–*120.*

Glasson C, Chapman K, James E. Fruit and vegetables should be targeted separately in health promotion programs: Differences in consumption levels, barriers, knowledge and stages of readiness for change. *Public Health Nutr.*, 2011;14(4):694-701.

Golan E, Stewart H, Kuchler F, Dong D. Can low-income Americans afford a healthy diet? *Amber Waves.* 2008;5:26-33.

Grigsby-Toussant DS, Zenk SN, Odoms-Young A, Ruggiero L, Moise I. Availability of commonly consumed and culturally specific fruits and vegetables in African-American and Latino neighborhoods. *J. Am. Diet. Assoc.*, 2010;110:746-752.

Gross SM, Pollock ED, Braun B. Family influence: Key to fruit and vegetable consumption among fourth- and fifth-grade students. *J. Nut. Educ. Behav.*, 2010;42(4):351-341.

Grutzmacher SG, Gross SM. Household food security and fruit and vegetable intake among low-income 4th graders. *J. Nut. Educ. Behav.* 2011;43(6):S14.

Gulliford MC, Nunes C and Rocke B. Food insecurity, weight control practices and body mass index. *Pub. Health Nutr.*, 2006;9(5):570-574.

Haldeman L, Gruber K, Ingram K. Determinants of food security and diet among rural and urban Latino/Hispanic immigrants. *J. Hunger. Environ. Nutr.*, 2008;2(4):67-83.

Hanson K, Andrews M. Rising Food Prices Take a Bite Out of Food Stamp Benefits. ERS bulletin No EIB-41. Economic Research Service, United States Department of Agriculture, 2008.

Havas S, Treiman K, Langenberg P, et al. Factors associated with fruit and vegetable consumption among women participating in WIC. *J. Am. Diet. Assoc.,* 1998;98:1141–*1148.*

Herman DR, Harrison GG, Afifi AA, Jenks E. Effect of a targeted subsidy on intake of fruits and vegetables among low-income women in the Special Supplemental Nutrition Program for Women, Infants, and Children. *Am. J. Public Health.* 2008;98(1):98-105.

Hildebrand DA, Shriver LH. A quantitative and qualitative approach to understanding fruit and vegetable availability in low-income African-American families with children enrolled in an urban head start program. *J. Am. Diet. Assoc.*, 2010;110(5):710-718.

Hoisington A, Schultz JA, Butkus S. Coping strategies and nutrition education needs among food pantry users. *J. Nutr. Educ. Behav.*, 2002;34(6):326-333.

Inglis V, Ball K, Crawford D. Socioeconomic variations in women's diets: What is the role of perceptions of the local food environment? *Epidemiology Comm.Health.* 2008;62(3):191-197.

Institute of Medicine. School Meals: Building Blocks for Healthy Children. Washington, DC: The National Academies Press, 2009.

Kaiser LL, Melgar-Quiñonez H, Lamp C, Sutherlin J, Johns M, Harwood J. Food security and nutritional outcomes of Latino preschoolers. *J. Am. Diet. Assoc.* 2,002;102:924-929.

Kaiser LL, Melgar-Quinonez H, Townsend MS, et al. Food insecurity and food supplies in Latino households with young children. *J. Nutr. Educ. Behav.* 2003;35:148-153.

Kamphuis CBM, Giskes K, De Bruijn GJ, Wendel-Vos W, Brug J, Van Lenthe FJ. Environmental determinants of fruit and vegetable consumption among adults: A systematic review. *Br J. Nutr.* October 2006;96(4):620-635.

Kendall A, Olson C, Frongillo E. Relationship of hunger and food insecurity to food availability and consumption. *J. Am. Diet. Assoc.* 1996;96:1019-1024.

Kendall A, Olson CM, Frongillo EA. Validation of the Radimer/Cornell measures of hunger and food insecurity. *J. Nutr.* 1995;125(11):2793-2801.

Kilanowski JF, Moore LC. Food security and dietary intake in Midwest migrant farmworker children. *J. Pediatr. Nurs.,* 2010;25(5):360-366.

Kropf ML, Holben DH, Holcomb JP, Anderson H. Food security status and produce intake and behaviors of Special Supplemental Nutrition Program for Women, Infants, and Children and Farmers' Market Nutrition Program participants. *J. Am. Diet. Assoc.*, 2007;107(11):1903-1908.

Lara M, Gamboa C, Kahramanian MI, Morales LS, Bautista DE. Acculturation and Latino health in the United States: A review of the literature and its sociopolitical context. *Annu. Rev of Public Health,* 2005;26:367-397.

Lorson BA, Melgar-Quinonez HR, Taylor CA. Correlates of fruit and vegetable intakes in US children. *J. Am. Diet. Assoc.*, 2009;109(3):474-478.

Lucan SC, Barg FK, Long JA. Promoters and barriers to fruit, vegetable, and fast-food consumption among urban, low-income African Americans:A qualitative approach. *Am. J. Public Health.*, 2010;100(4):631-635.

Maillot M, Darmon N, Drewnowski A. Are the lowest-cost healthful food plans culturally and socially acceptable? *Public Health Nutr.,* November 2010;13(8):1178-1185.

Matheson DM, Varady J, Varady A, et al. Household food security and nutritional status of Hispanic children in the fifth grade. *Am. J. Clin. Nutr.*, 2002;76(1):210-217.

Mathews L, Morris MN, Schneider J, Goto K. The relationship between food security and poor health among female WIC participants. *J. Hunger Environ. Nutr.*, 2010;5(1):85-99.

Mello JA, Gans KM, Risica PM, et al. How is food insecurity associated with dietary behaviors? An analysis with low-income, ethnically diverse participants in a nutrition intervention study. *J. Am. Diet. Assoc.*, 2010;110(12):1906-1911.

Monsivais P, Aggarwal A, Drewnowski A. Are socio-economic disparities in diet quality explained by diet cost? *J. Epidemiol. Comm. Health.,* 2010.

Monsivais P, Drewnowski A. The rising cost of low-energy-density foods. *J. Am. Diet. Assoc.,* December 2007;107(12):2071-2076.

Monsivais P, Drewnowski A. Lower-energy-density diets are associated with higher monetary costs per kilocalorie and are consumed by women of higher socioeconomic status. *J. Am. Diet. Assoc.,* May 2009;109(5):814-822.

Munoz K, Krebs-Smith S, Ballard-Barbash R, et al. Children and adolescents don't follow the food pyramid. *Nutr. Res. Newsletter,* Nov/Dec 1997;16(11/12):114-116.

Neuhouser ML, Thompson B, Coronado GD, Solomon CC. Higher fat intake and lower fruit and vegetables intakes are associated with greater acculturation among Mexicans living in Washington State. *J. Am. Diet. Assoc.,* 2004;104(1):51-57.

Nord M, Bickel G. Measuring Children's Food Security in U.S. Households, 1995–1999. Food Assistance and Nutrition Research Report No. 25. Washington, DC: US Department of Agriculture, Food and Nutrition Service and Economic Research Service; 2002.http://www.ers.usda.gov/ publications/fanrr25/fanrr25.pdf. Accessed June 29, 2011.

Nord M, Bickel G. Estimating the prevalence of children's hunger from the Current Population Survey Food Security Supplement. In: Andrews M, Prell M, editors. Second Food Security Measurement and Research Conference, Volume II: Papers. Food Assistance and Nutrition Research Report 11–2:31–49. 2001. Washington, DC: Economic Research Service, USDA.

Nord M, Hopwood H. Recent advances provide improved tools for measuring children's food security. *J. Nutr.*, 2007;137(3):533–536.

Nord M, Coleman-Jensen A, Andrews M, Carlson S. Household food insecurity in the United States, 2009. *Economic Research Report No. ERR-108,* Economic Research Service, United States Department of Agriculture, 2010.

Nöthlings U, Schulze MB, Weikert C, et al. Intake of vegetables, legumes, and fruit, and risk for all-cause, cardiovascular, and cancer mortality in a European diabetic population. *J. Nutr.,* April 2008;138(4):775-781.

Oberhosler CA, Tuttle CR. Assessment of household food security among food stamp recipient families in Maryland. *Am. J. Public Health.*, May 2004;94(5):790-795.

Olson CM. Food insecurity in women: A recipe for unhealthy trade-offs. *Top. Clin. Nutr.*, 2005;20(4):321-328.

Patterson, RE, Haines PS, Popkin BM. Diet quality index: capturing a multidimensional behavior. *J. Am. Diet. Assoc.*, 1994;94(1):57-64.

Peterson SL, Dodd KM, Kim K, Roth SL. Food cost perceptions and food purchasing practices of uninsured, low-income, rural adults. *J. Hunger. Environ. Nutr.,* 2010;5(1):41-55.

Raedeke M. Food security, nutrition and health of food pantry participants. Dissertation submitted to University of Missouri - Columbia, 2007, 125 pages; pub no. 3322737. http://gateway.proquest. com/openurl% 3furl_ver=Z39.88-2004% 26res_dat=xri:pqdiss%26rft_val_fmt=info:ofi/fmt:kev:mtx:dissertation%26rft_dat=xri:pqdiss:3322737. Accessed July 30, 2011.

Renzaho A, Kumanyika S, Tucker K. Family functioning, parental psychological distress, child behavioral problems, socio-economic disadvantage and fruit and vegetable consumption among 4–12 year-old Victorians, Australia. *Health Promot Int.* September 2011;26(3):263-275.

Smith C, Richards R. Dietary intake, overweight status, and perceptions of food insecurity among homeless Minnesotan youth. *Am. J. Hum. Biol.*, September/October 2008;20(5):550-563.

Speirs KE, Braun B, Zoumenou V, et al. Grandmothers' involvement in preschool-aged children's consumption of fruits and vegetables. *Infant. Child Adolesc. Nutr.*, December 2009;1(6):332-337.

Stuff JE, Casey PH, Szeto KL, et al. Household food insecurity is associated with adult health status. *J. Nutr.,* September 2004;132(9):2330-2335.

Stuff JE, LaCour M, Du X, et al. The prevalence of food insecurity and associated factors among households with children in head start programs in Houston, Texas and Birmingham, Alabama. *Race, Gender and Class*, 2009;16(3-4):31-47.

Tarasuk V, McIntyre L, Li J. Low-income women's dietary intakes are sensitive to the depletion of household resources in one month. *Comm. Health*, 2007:137(8)1980-1987.

Tingay RS, Tan CJ, Tan NC, et al. Food insecurity and low income in an English inner city. *J. Public Health Med.*, June 2003;25(2):156-159.

Townsend MS, Kaiser LL, Allen LH, Joy AB, Murphy SP. Selecting items for a food behavior checklist for a limited–resource audience. *J. Nutr. Educ. Behav.,* March/April 2003;35(2):69-77.

Townsend MS, Peerson J, Love B, Achterberg C, Murphy SP. Food insecurity is positively related to overweight in women. *J. Nutr.*, 2001;131:1738-45.

Volpe R, Liebtag R. Food CPI and Expenditures: Analysis and Forecasts of the CPI for food. Economic Research Service Briefing Room, 2011.

Webber CB, Sobal J, Dollahite JS. Shopping for fruits and vegetables: Food and retail qualities of importance to low-income households at the grocery store. *Appetite.* 2010;54(2):297-303.

Widome R, Neumark-Sztainer D, Hannan PJ, Haines J, Story M. Eating when there is not enough to eat: Eating behaviors and perceptions of food among food-insecure youths. *Am. J. Public Health*, 2009;99(5):822-828.

Wilde P, Ranney C. *A Monthly Cycle in Food Expenditure and Intake by Participants in the U.S. Food Stamp Program.* Discussion Paper no. 1163-98, Institute for Research on Poverty, University of Madison-Wisconsin, 1998.

Wilde PE, Peterman JN. Individual weight change is associated with household food security status. *J. Nutr.*, 2006;136:1395-1400.

Zenk SN, Schulz AJ, Hollis-Neely T, et al. Fruit and vegetable intake in African Americans income and store characteristics. *Am. J. Prev. Med.*, 2005;29(1):1-9.

In: Vegetable Consumption and Health: New Research
Editors: Claudia Wilson and Melinda Morree
ISBN: 978-1-62100-941-2

Chapter 2

QUALITY CONTROL FOR PESTICE RESIDUES IN OLIVES AND OLIVE OIL

Antonio Ruiz-Medina* and Eulogio J. Llorent-Martínez
Department of Physical and Analytical Chemistry,
Faculty of Experimental Sciences, University of Jaén,
Campus Las Lagunillas, Jaén, Spain

ABSTRACT

Olive oil is a product of great importance in the sustainable economy of important regions from the main olive oil producers in the world, Spain, Italy and Greece. Due to the facts that virgin olive oil production has increased in recent years and that it is being exported to different countries, exhaustive quality controls are required. The application of phytosanitary products is one of the main employed procedures to solve the problems of plagues and diseases in olive groves. As a result, there is an increasing unease related to the possible presence of residues from these products in the olive-derived foods. Recent studies have shown that these residues can be found in olives and olive oil (mainly insecticides, fungicides and herbicides) due to the lipophilic nature of the used plaguicides. Different regulations regarding maximum residue limits (MRLs) in table olives and olive oil have been established by the European Union and the Codex Alimentarius of the Food and Agriculture Organization of the United Nations; in addition, new regulations will be established in following years. However, the detected levels of all these phytosanitary products are usually below the MRLs established.

A wide range of pesticides is used by olive farmers for pest management and vector control in agricultural areas. Sometimes, farmers use these compounds without full understanding of their impact on human health and the environment. Although the inhalation, dermal and oral routes of exposure are the most common, pesticide residues in food and water may add to indirect exposures in the general population. This constitutes a risk of these pesticides being incorporated in both: (a) rivers and reservoirs with the soil that is eroded in heavy rains, polluting surface waters, etc.; and (b) olives and, consequently, olive oil.

* Tel: (+34)953-212759; Fax: (+34)953-212940; E-mail: anruiz@ujaen.es.

There are alternative methods available for the analysis of pesticides in different kind of samples. However, the common methods of analysis for their determination are Gas Chromatography (GC) and Liquid Chromatography (LC). GC is usually the chosen technique due to the high separation efficiency and compatibility with a wide range of detection techniques. Our research group has performed thorough investigation over the analysis of pesticides in soils, olive fruits and virgin olive oils. In particular, we have developed different GC analytical methods with mass spectrometric detection for the analysis of all the main pesticides used in olive groves. In this way, sensitive and reliable procedures can be implemented for the quality control of table olives and olive oils in the industry. These methodologies will be briefly described in this chapter.

1. Introduction

Nowadays, olive groves represent one of the main plantations in the countries of the Mediterranean Basin (the adjoining coastal areas of southeastern Europe, western Asia and northern Africa), especially in the South and Center of Spain and Italy, in Greece, Turkey, Tunisia and Morocco [1]. The present situation of olive groves is the result of a slow and continuous development of the different civilizations who inhabited Mediterranean coastal areas and the inner lands of Middle East. The economic significance of olive oils varies among the producer countries and can be crucial in some of the mentioned countries, where the olive oil sector represents a high percentage of the economic activity. For instance, in Spain, more than half a million farmers work in olive groves. In other countries, such as Tunisia, olive oil is more than just goods; it is a strategic product for exportation activities, as the country has obtained valuable subsidizations from the European Union.

The olive is one of the plants most often cited in literature and probably the oldest one in historic publications. At first sight, olive oil does not seem to be so important when global statistical data in terms of production and consumption are observed. However, olive oil really represents a remarkable percentage of worldwide trading because its value per unit of product is significantly higher than that one of other edible oils (soybean, corn, sunflower, etc). The beneficial effects of consuming olive oil are backed by lengthy, painstaking scientific research.

Fats and oils have a common denominator in the energy value (9 calories per gram, approximately) but the metabolism of each different group greatly differs from the rest. Olive oil contains a series of compounds that are very beneficial to most functions of the human body and its biological and therapeutic value is related in many aspects to its chemical structure, specially virgin olive oil, which is a natural product obtained from the olive fruit (Olea Europaea) using solely mechanical or physical means. The fact that oil extraction is solvent-free and natural antioxidants are maintained in the oil is reflected in the high nutritional and economic value of this product. As a result, consumer's demand of this product has increased worldwide and it is the main ingredient of the Mediterranean diet.

2. Composition and Health Benefits of Olive Oil

Olive oil is composed mainly of triglycerides (98-99% of the olive oil) and contains small quantities of free fatty acids (FFA), being the proportion of FFA variable and related to the degree of hydrolysis of the triglycerides. The composition of FFA in the oil depends on the variety of the olive tree, climatic conditions and geographical localization of the grove. Both the International Olive Council (IOC) and the Codex Alimentarius Comission have established maximum and minimum percentages for each fatty acid in the composition of the olive and pomace-olive oils. In general, olive oil is basically composed of mono-insaturated fatty acids. Regarding the degree of insaturation, FFA composition is as follows: 72% mono-insaturated, 14% poli-insaturated and 14% saturated.

There are also minor components in olive oil, which are specific markers of its physico-chemical authenticity and they also add unique sensory and biological characteristics:

- Squalene is the major olive oil terpenoid hydrocarbon (300-700 mg L^{-1}), whereas β-carotene, biological precursor of vitamin A, is found in small quantities (few mg L^{-1}).
- Triterpenoids alcohols (24-methylenecycloartanol, cycloartenol, α-amirine and β-amirine) are especially important from the biological point of view. Eritrodiol is also important from the analytical perspective, because it can be used to detect the presence of pomace-olive oil.
- Sterols can be used to construct a fingerprint in order to authenticate the olive oil, specifically using the β-sitosterol content, which represents around 93% of the total content of sterols.
- Tocopherols, especially α-tocopherol or vitamin E (150-300 mg L^{-1}), are important antioxidants.
- Phenolic compounds, which contribute to the characteristic flavor of olive oil and increase the antioxidant properties of the oil.
- One hundred aromatic compounds are also present, approximately, being the exact chemical composition dependent on the variety, climatic conditions and quality of the oil.

Virgin olive oil is the most digestible of the edible fats and it helps to assimilate vitamins A, D and K. It contains essential acids that cannot be produced by our own bodies, slows down the aging process and helps bile, liver and intestinal functions. It is noteworthy that olive oil has a beneficial effect in the dietary treatment of diabetes.

In addition, it helps to control blood pressure and increases the bone mass. It is believed that olive oil has a favorable effect on the development of the central nervous and vascular systems, in brain development, as well as in normal child development [1,2].

The human body easily absorbs this type of oil. This means that the body absorbs the good ingredients such as vitamin E and phenols, which have anti-oxidizing properties and prevent the oxidization of fatty tissue. Olive oil is not only easy to digest but it also helps the digestion of other fatty substances because it helps the secretions of the peptic system and stimulates the pancreatic enzyme lipase. Moreover, its consumption has a very positive effect on blood cholesterol because it limits the oxidizing of bad cholesterol (cause of heart disease).

Olive oil, as any fatty substance, deteriorates during the frying process especially if it is used over and over and if the frying temperature is very high. High temperature destroys the good ingredients of any oil while it creates harmful agents for the liver, the arteries and the heart. However, it is important to take into consideration that these harmful agents are less likely to be created in olive oil than in all other known vegetable oils because of their different composition. Olive oil contains a high percentage of oleic acid, which is much more resistant to oxidization than polyunsaturated acids, which are found in large amounts in seed oils. In addition, it contains natural anti-oxidizing agents, therefore making olive oil the most stable fat and it stands up well to high frying temperatures. Hence, the digestibility of olive oil is not affected when it is heated.

3. Olive Oil Elaboration and Classification

The technology for olive oil extraction, called elaiotechnic, is the fundamental basis for obtaining high-quality virgin olive oil (extra virgin). The main steps required for the elaboration of virgin olive oil follow.

Harvest of Olives

The harvest of the olives could be understood as an independent activity from the elaboration of the oil. However, the characteristics of the oil are highly influenced by the harvest time and method employed.

Olives must be picked at the moment of optimum ripeness, where the fruit presents the maximum content of oil and the best characteristics. Olives reach their ripeness in autumn and picking starts at the end of November, lasting up to February or March.

The methods to harvest the olives have not changed much from the ancient times. The methods used should not damage the fruit and should avoid breaking of boughs or shoots. The high-quality olive oil is obtained by "milking" the olives into a sack tied around the harvester's waist (using ladders for the highest boughs) and extending canvases at the foot of the trees, where the olives will fall when the tree is beaten (using flexible poles). Recent methods make use of harvester machines (shakers) that generate the vibration on the tree for the falling of the fruit. This vibration machines can be small vibrators operated by the farmer in the required boughs or fully-equipped tractors, with vibration units for the whole trunk of the tree and an umbrella to pick the olives.

Harvest by hand is impossible in olive trees of 4-5 meters high, even with the use of ladders. In general, the olives are picked directly from the ground after they fall down in a natural way when they reach ripeness. When this happens, weeds should be completely eliminated from the zone in order to make it easier the picking. Anyway, the quality of the olive oil obtained from this olives is poor, because organoleptics flaws, such as soil flavor, are very evident.

Washing

Traditionally, agricultural workers have cleaned the fruit in the fields, by means of sieves. But this cleaning is not complete and the fruit goes into the olive-oil mill with a great quantity of impurities, leaves, branches, mud, etc., which is necessary to eliminate.

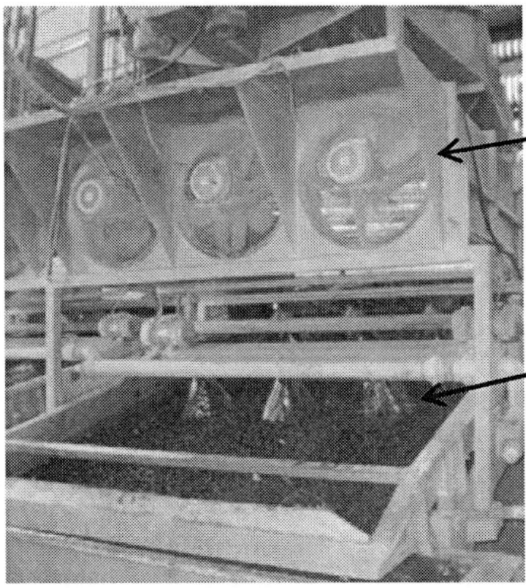

Figure 1. Cleaning steps for olive fruits.

Therefore, for this purpose, cleaners that use air current or shaking sieves are used to eliminate leaves, branches and other impurities lighter than the fruits. In addition, washing devices are employed to eliminate heavier impurities, such as stones or dust. In the next figure, both cleaning steps, the one with the air for light impurities and the other one by washing for heavy impurities, are shown.

Once the fruit has been cleaned and weighed, it is stored in hoppers until it can be crushed. The storage period must be as short as possible in order to avoid alterations, which would produce oils with a higher degree of acidity, lower stability and worse flavor.

Preparation

The process of releasing the oil from the plant tissue begins by milling the olives to tear the flesh cells in order to let the oil run out of the vacuoles. This is followed by stirring the olive paste to permit the formation of large drops of oil and to break up the oil–water emulsion. In the so-called "dual-phase decanters" the oil is then separated by direct continuous centrifugation from the pomace, which consists of vegetable matter and water. The yield of oil varies from 80 to 90% of the total oil content of the olives, because the oil in the olive paste is only partially free to escape and part of it remains in the unbroken cells or is trapped in the tissues of the cytoplasm, or is emulsified in the aqueous phase.

After the extraction of virgin olive oil from the olives, the remaining paste is called pomace and still contains a small quantity (2-6%) of oil that can only be extracted with chemical solvents. This is done in specialized chemical plants, not in the olive oil mills and the obtained oil is called pomace oil.

The limit of FFA in olive oil for direct consumption is 2%. Virgin olive oils with higher content are called "lampantes" and must be refined prior to consumption. The components to be removed are all those ones that are detrimental to the flavor, color and stability of the oil, mainly FFA, phosphoacylglycerols, pigments, volatiles and contaminants. The standard processes used are chemical and physical refining. The main difference between both processes is that chemical refining procedure includes caustic soda treatment to neutralize the oil while, following physical refining, FFA are eliminated by distillation during deodorization. Physical refining reduces the loss of neutral oil, minimizes pollution and enables recovery of high quality FFA. Nevertheless, not all oils can be physically refined.

Taking into account all the procedure in order to obtain the oil, edible olive oil is marketed in accordance with the following designations and definitions [3]:

a) *Virgin olive oil:* it is the oil obtained from the fruit of the olive tree solely by mechanical or other physical means under conditions, particularly thermal conditions, that do not lead to alterations in the oil, and which have not undergone any treatment other than washing, decantation, centrifugation and filtration. The virgin olive oils that are fit for consumption are extra virgin olive oil and virgin olive oil, presenting a free acidity, expressed as oleic acid, of not more than 0.8 and 2 grams per 100 grams, respectively. They also have to fulfil different quality criteria that, according to the IOC, include good organoleptic characteristics (taste and aroma) and low peroxide value.
b) *Olive oil:* it is the oil consisting of a blend (approximately 80:20 v:v) of refined olive oil and virgin olive oil fit for consumption as they are. It has a free acidity, expressed as oleic acid, of not more than 1 gram per 100 grams and its other characteristics correspond to those fixed for this category in this standard.
c) *Olive pomace oil:* it is the oil obtained by treating olive pomace with solvents or other physical treatments, to the exclusion of oils obtained by re-esterification processes and of any mixture with oils of other kinds. The marketed olive pomace oil is the oil comprising the blend (approximately 80:20 v:v) of refined olive-pomace oil and virgin olive oil fit for consumption as they are. It has a free acidity (expressed as oleic acid) of not more than 1 gram per 100 grams.

Chemical processing may improve high acidity olive oil and make it edible; however, it takes away some extremely valuable ingredients such as vitamins and phenols. As a result, processed olive oil (refined) lacks the desirable properties and characteristics that can be found in abundance in virgin olive oil.

4. Plagues and Pesticides

The attacks of pests and diseases and the presence of weeds make it necessary to apply pesticides to olive trees to ensure crop protection. The denomination pesticides (or plaguicides) include a wide variety of products that are very different in their chemical composition and characteristics. A plaguicide can be described as a substance (or formulation containing at least one of them) that presents any of the following uses:

- Fight agents that can be harmful for the crops or prevent the potential effects of these agents.
- Control or regulate the vegetable production.
- Protect the vegetable production, including woods.

- Destruct weeds.
- Destruct part of the vegetables or prevent undesirable growths.
- Destruct or prevent the action of potentially harmful organisms different to the ones that attack plants.

Taking into account the specific action of the plaguicides, different classifications can be made, being the decimal classification one of the most frequently used:

- Insecticides are used against insects and they include ovicides and larvicides (against eggs and larvae of insects, respectively). Nearly all insecticides have the potential to significantly alter ecosystems, being many of them toxic to humans.
- Acaricides kill members of the Acari group, which includes ticks and mites.
- Fungicides are chemical compounds or biological organisms used to kill or inhibit fungi or fungal spores.
- Nematocides, disinfectants and fumigants in general, used to kill parasitic nematodes.
- Herbicides are used to kill unwanted plants while leaving the desired crop relatively unharmed.
- Phytoregulators and similar products can be used to improve the potential of the trees.
- Molusquicides and rodenticides are used to control molluscs (slugs and snails) and rodents pests.
- Post-harvest pesticides and seeds.
- Protectors of woods, fibers and derivatives.
- Other specific plaguicides.

Laboratory studies show that pesticides can cause health problems, such as birth defects, nerve damage, cancer, and other effects that might occur over a long period of time. However, these effects depend on how toxic the pesticide is and how much of it is consumed. Some pesticides also pose unique health risks to children. For these reasons, the governments carefully regulate pesticides to ensure that their use does not pose unreasonable risks to human health or the environment.

The mechanisms of action of the plaguicides over the organism are very different depending on their chemical composition. These mechanisms are well-known for some of them, even at the molecular level. However, they are completely unknown for some others. Even among pesticides from the same family, some of them can be classified as scarcely toxic while others are very toxic. As a result, it is difficult to establish general rules when dealing with the toxicity of plaguicides.

Many organochlorine compounds affect the central nervous system, the liver and the kidneys. They accumulate in adipose tissues and are slowly eliminated. Organophosphorus and carbamate compounds affect the central nervous system too, inhibiting the acetylcholinesterase enzyme.

Environmental control allows to make an estimation of the exposing risk taking into account the levels of the toxic compound(s) in the air. However, this option is only useful when the compound is only toxic by inhalation. In the case of plaguicides, it is more interesting to calculate the real exposing risk using biological control, because pesticides can enter the organism through other channels different to inhalation. The biological control may consist in the direct determination of the plaguicide and metabolites in biological fluids, such as the determination of different organochlorine pesticides in urine. The obtained levels are compared with established Biological Exposure Index (BEI), which are values used for guidance to assess biological monitoring results.

The use of pesticides is the main way to fight against pests and plagues in olive groves. The plagues and diseases of the olive tree have changed little since ancient times. The most important ones are the olive fruit fly and the olive moth. The third one in importance is black scale, which appeared around the sixties. These plagues will be briefly described.

Olive Fruit Fly

The olive fruit fly (*Bactrocera oleae*) is a species of fruit fly which belongs to the Dacinae subfamily. It is a kind of phytophagous species, whose larvae feed on the fruit of olive trees, hence the common name. It is considered the most serious pest in the cultivation of olives. It is found throughout the Mediterranean Basin and in South Africa. Since the late 1990s it has also been present in California and has possibly spread throughout the area of olive cultivation in the Nearctic region.

The damage caused by the olive fruit fly can be quantitative and qualitative. In most cases, the greatest damage occurs as the fruit begins to soften and turn color, from September to November. The adult female can lay 50 to 400 eggs, generally one in each fruit. Olive fly eggs are small and difficult to see, embedded under the fruit surface. The tiny larvae hatching from the eggs are also quite difficult to see until they feed for a while and get larger. The first damage sign is an oviposition "sting" on the fruit surface. This looks like a small indentation or lump on the surface. Sometimes there is discoloration. While feeding, the larvae tunnel through the fruit, destroying the pulp and allowing entry of secondary infestation of bacteria and fungi that rot the fruit and greatly lower the quality of oil. The oil's FFA level ("acidity") increases considerably. If the damage is extensive enough, it may cause premature fruit drop. In areas of the world where the olive fruit fly is established and not controlled, its damage has been responsible for losses of up to 80% of oil value because of lower quantity and quality, and in some varieties of table olives, this pest is capable of destroying 100% of the crop.

The chemical battle against the olive fruit fly can be implemented against larvae by using preventive treatments against adults. The treatments are carried out by spraying the olive trees with insecticides, such as dimethoate, which is the most common due to its effectiveness and relatively low cost.

Olive Moth

Olive moth or olive kernel borer *(Prays oleae Bern)* is an important insect in the Mediterranean Basin and the United States and the second plague in importance. Three yearly generations are typical of this species. Each one is associated during the larval stage to different parts of the host. First generation larvae attack the flower buds, the second generation larvae grow inside the olive stone kernel and the third generation larvae are leaf mine. The damage (leaf drop) done by the leaf or third generation is seldom serious. On the contrary, damage caused by flower generation can be important. The larvae directly destroy the flowers or cause the abortion of the flower bunches covered by silken threads spun by the larvae when passing from one bud to the next. The fruit generation larvae cause the premature drop of the fruits when they bore the kernel of the olive fruit or later when they try to vacate the fruit to pupate. If the fall of the fruit takes place in June, the tree compensates this effect by increasing the size of the remaining fruits. However, a great reduction in the yielding and quality of the oil would be caused if the falling occurs in September.

There are two moments of action to fight this plague, at the beginning of the flowering (the period when the larvae are outside the fruit) or when the larvae are introducing themselves in the fruit. The plaguicides usually employed for the control of the olive moth are dimethoate and formothion, although others such as carbaryl can be used too.

Black Scale

Black scale (*Saissetia oleae*) is very common in all Mediterranean countries where olive tree is cultivated. This plague is caused by small black insects that cover the plants' leaves and stems. They sap the nutrients from the tree and excrete sticky, shiny honeydew on leaves of infested trees. At first, affected trees and leaves glisten and then become sooty and black in appearance as sooty mold fungus grows on the honeydew. Infestations reduce vigor and productivity of the tree, because the plant is denied the necessary sunlight. Continuous feeding reduces bloom the following year.

For controlling small amounts of black scale, it is possible to simply brush it off the stem or leaf with a toothbrush or knife. However, for larger infestations, chemical treatment could be required, although spraying oil on the plant can suffocate the pest sometimes. Some of the pesticides that can be used against black scale are dimethoate, diazinon and carbaryl.

5. Pesticides Analyzed in Olive Oil

As a result of the cited plagues, it is necessary to introduce the use of insecticides in the olive groves not only for the treatment of established plagues, but also for prevention. In addition, herbicides are required to control the growth of weeds. The absence of weeds in the soil around the olive tree presents two major benefits: the weeds do not waste water resources for the olive trees and the harvest of olives from the soil is easier when they naturally fall down from the tree.

In the following Tables (Tables 1-4), the pesticides that are usually employed in the Spanish olive groves are shown, classified by chemical families (organochlorines, orgahophosphorous, triazines, phtalimides, carbamates and phenylureas). In these Tables, not only plaguicides used in olive trees are shown, but also others that are employed in plantations close to olive groves and can be found in the olive oil. In addition, the use of some pesticides such as DDT or simazine is forbidden, but they are very persistent and they have to be analyzed in order to ensure the absence of their residues in the food.

Organochlorine pesticides are insecticides with a highly stable, low volatile, lipophilic nature, consequently exhibiting considerable environmental persistence with a tendency to bioaccumulate, especially in foodstuffs with a high fat content [4]. With the introduction of new regulations against the use of organochlorines, other insecticides replaced them, such as the carbamate carbaryl and the organophosphorus, which are less stable in the environment [5]. Triazines, phenylurea diuron and phenylether oxyfluorphen are herbicides too, whereas phtalimides act as fungicides.

The water solubility (W.S.) at 25 °C and the $K_{O/W}$ value are also presented in Tables 1-4. The $K_{O/W}$ value is the partition coefficient between octanol and water, and its logarithm is an indication of fat solubility of the plaguicide. A high value of the coefficient $K_{O/W}$ for a particular plaguicide indicates that its solubility in water is low; hence, this plaguicide would be fat-soluble and there would be risks of bio-accumulation in fatty tissues. It has been demonstrated that fat-soluble pesticides tend to concentrate in olive oil during its production and extraction from the olives. For this reason, higher concentration levels of fat-soluble plaguicides are expected in the oil than in the olives from which the oil was produced. On the other hand, polar pesticides do not tend to preconcentrate in olive oil and their concentration is lower.

Table 1. Organochlorines

Plaguicide	Structure	W.S. (mg L^{-1})	$K_{O/W}$ 25°C
α-HCH	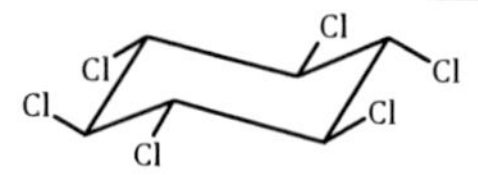	1.9	3.82
Lindane (γ-HCH)	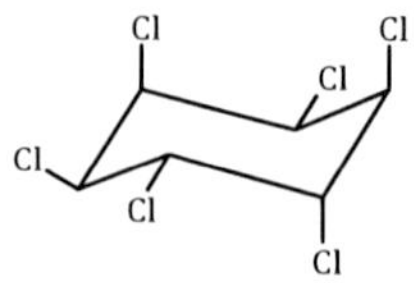	8.5	3.69
Heptachlor	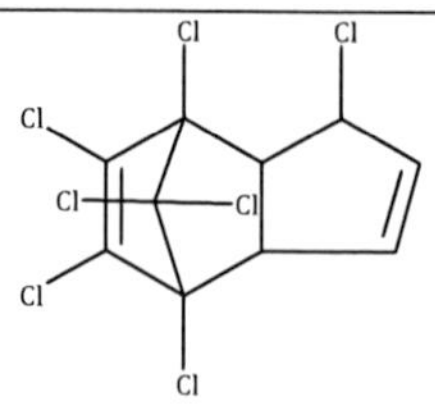	0.06	5.44
Aldrin	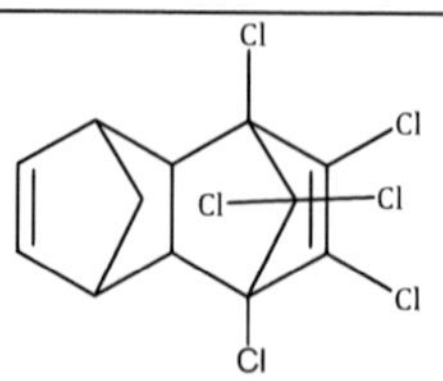	0.03	6.50

Plaguicide	Structure	W.S. (mg L^{-1})	$K_{O/W}$ 25°C
Dieldrin	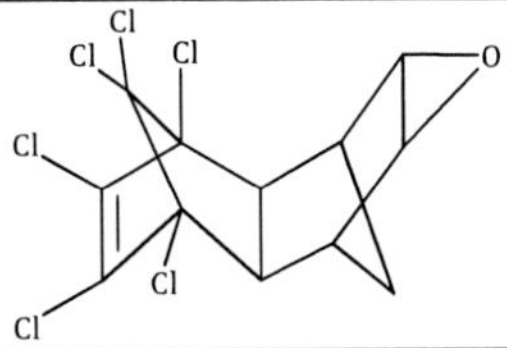	0.14	3.70
α-Endosulfan	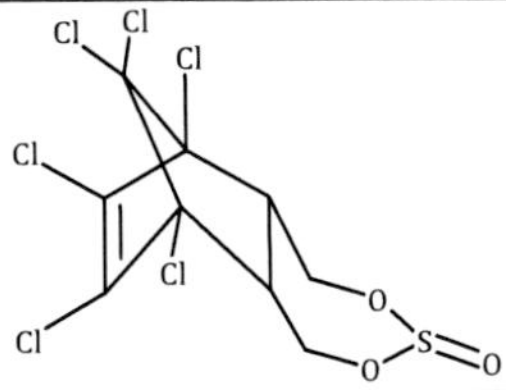	0.32	4.74
β-Endosulfan	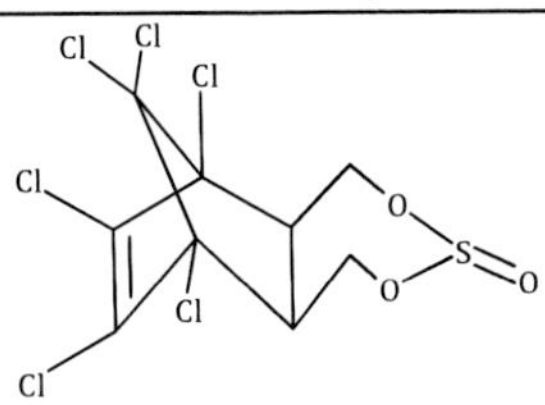	0.33	4.79
Endosulfan sulfate	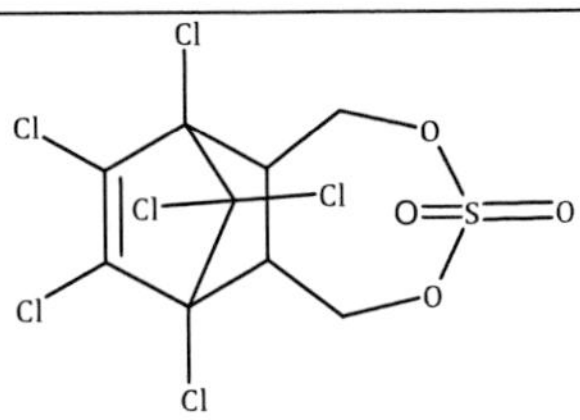	0.48	3.66
Endrin	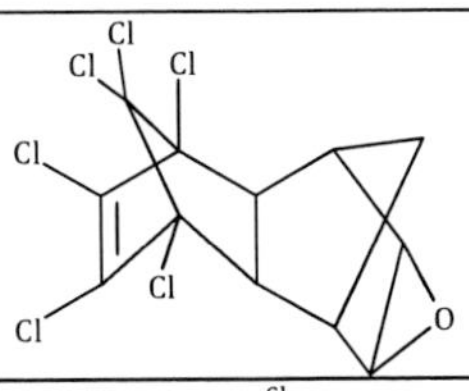	0.24	3.20
DDT	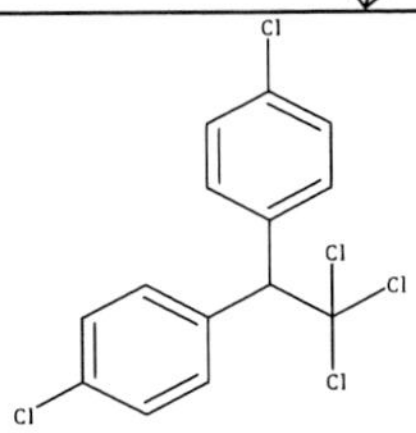	Not appreciable	6.91
DDD	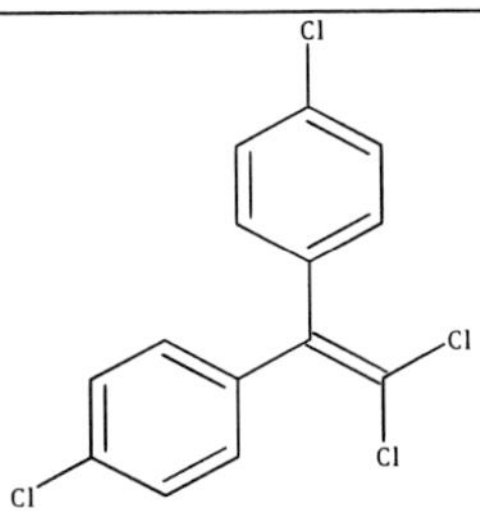	--	--

Monitoring pesticide residues in olive oil and olives is therefore of great interest to ensure food safety related to their use. The development of multi-residue methods, which allow proper control of a large number of pesticides in the same sale, is required. These methods need to present a high sensitivity in order to be able to analyze the samples at the legislated MRLs.

The analysis of pesticide residues in olive oil is very challenging, because of the inherent complexity of the matrix. As a result, it is necessary to extract the pesticide fraction from the whole matrix to isolate the compounds that will be analyzed. Taking into account that some pesticides are fat-soluble, it is difficult to completely separate them from the matrix. Hence, a clean-up step is required after the extraction procedure.

Table 2. Organophosphorus

Plaguicide	Structure	W.S. (mg L^{-1})	$K_{O/W}$ 25°C
Dimethoate	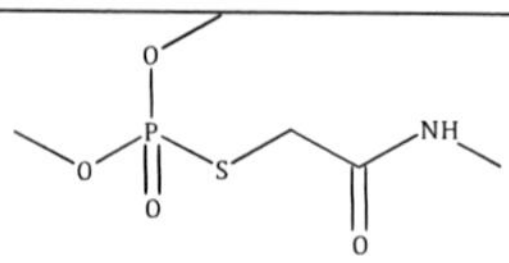	23.3	0.70
Diazinon	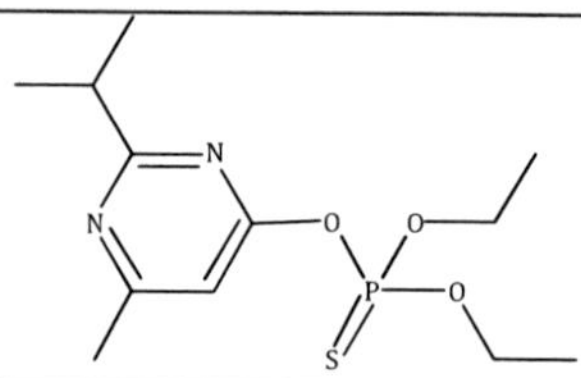	60	3.30
Formothion	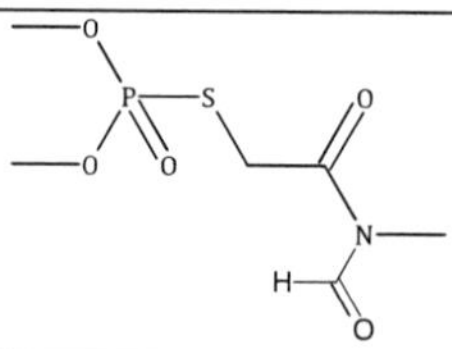	2600	1.48
Chlorpyrifos	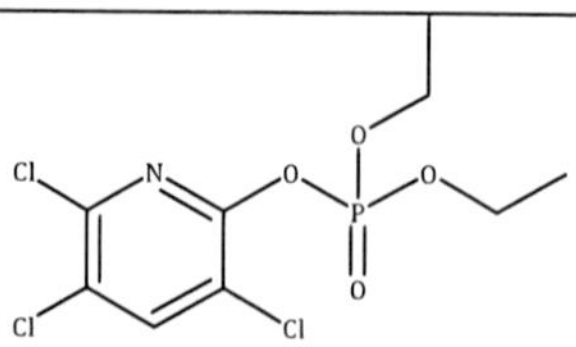	1.4	4.96
Chlorpyrifos-methyl	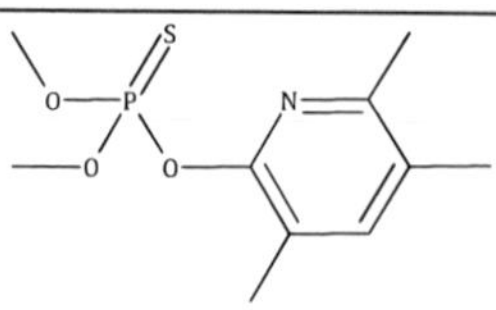	2.6	4.24
Pirimiphos-methyl	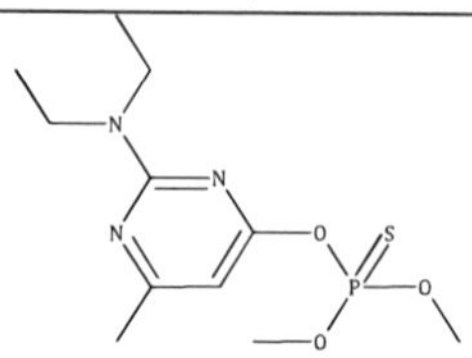	11	4.20

Plaguicide	Structure	W.S. (mg L^{-1})	$K_{O/W}$ 25°C
Malathion	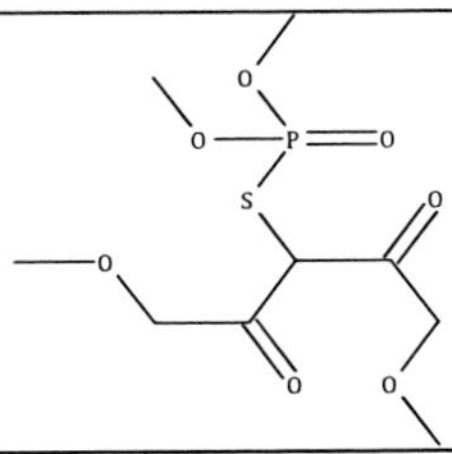	145	2.75
Fenitrothion	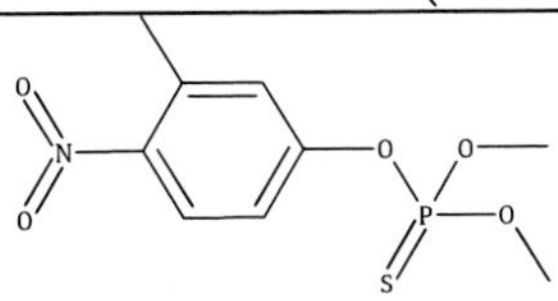	14	3.43
Methidathion	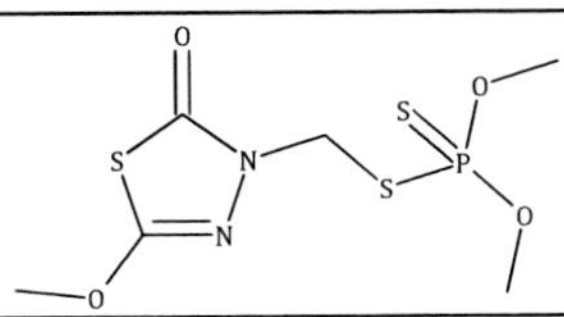	200	2.20

Table 3. Triazines

Plaguicide	Structure	W.S. (mg L^{-1})	$K_{O/W}$ 25°C
Simazine	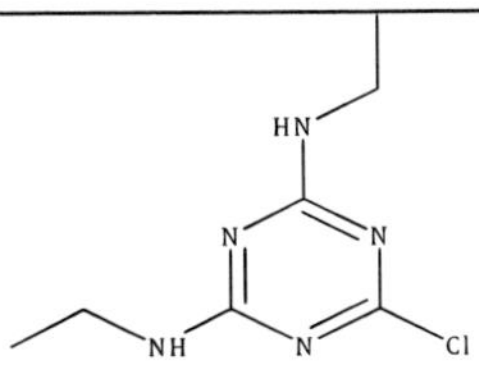	1.3	2.10
Atrazine	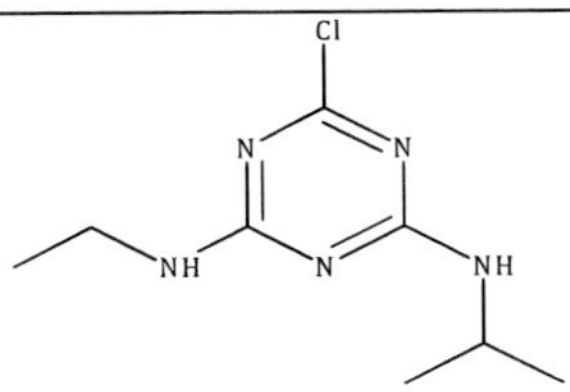	33	2.50
Trietazine	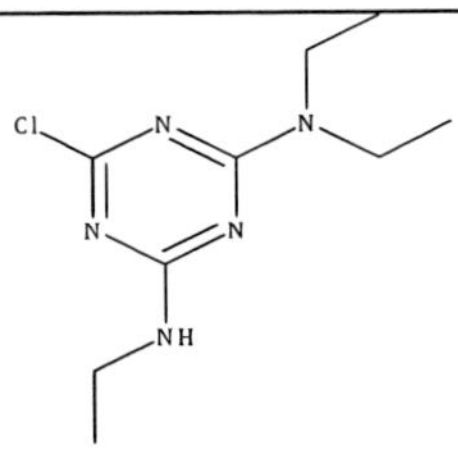	20	3.34
Terbuthylazine	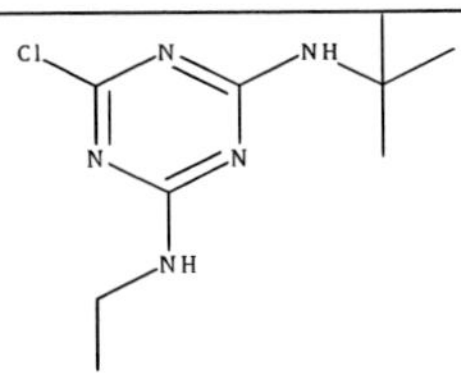	8.5	3.21

Table 4. Other families

Plaguicide	Structure	W.S. (mg L^{-1})	$K_{O/W}$ 25°C
Terbutrine	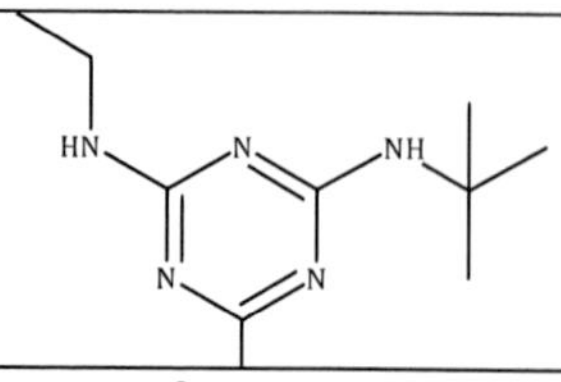	22	3.65
Diuron[1]	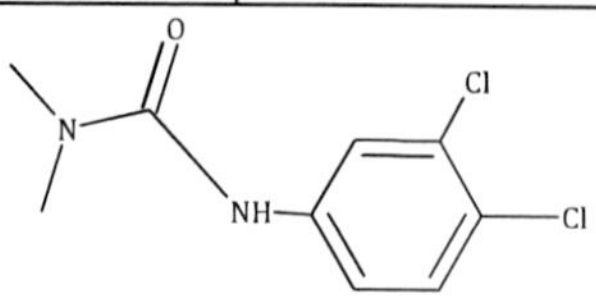	36.4	2.85
Carbaryl[2]	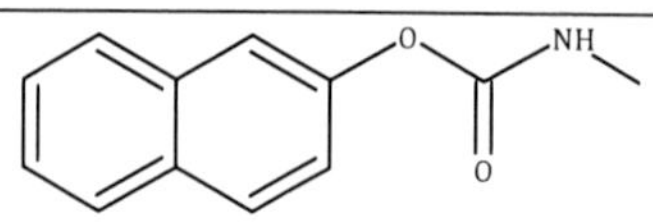	120	1.59
Folpet[3]	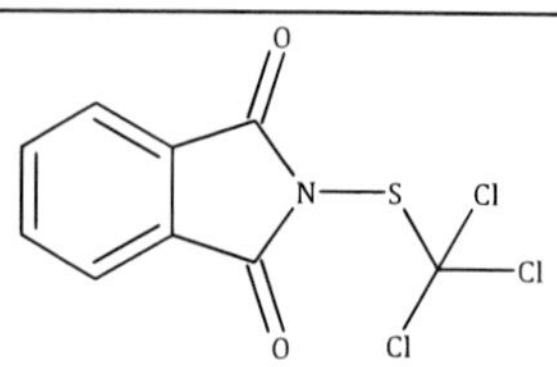	0.8	3.11
Captan[3]	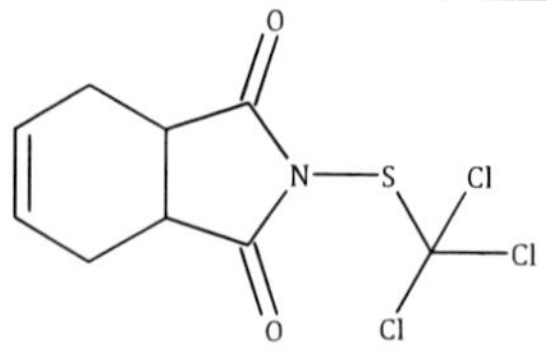	3.3	2.80
Oxyfluorfen[4]	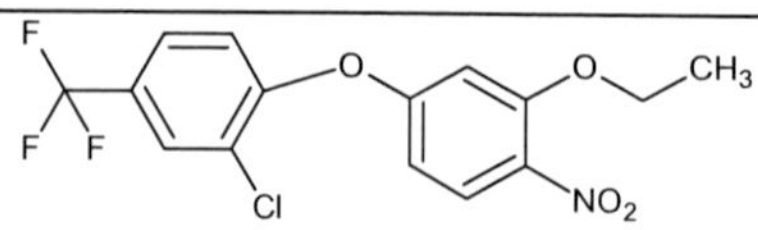	0.116	4.86

[1] Phenylurea; [2] Carbamate; [3] Phthalimide; [4] Phenylether.

6. Sample Preparation and Determination by Gas Chromatography

The first step required in the analysis of plaguicides is to separate the analytes from the matrix and other interfering compounds, therefore isolating the plaguicides from the rest of the sample. This separation includes extraction, preconcentration and clean-up steps, although sometimes they can be performed at the same time [6,7].

This part of the analysis is critical, because the final results will be completely related to the success of the separation process. The sample has to come into contact with an extractant (solid, liquid or supercritical fluid) in optimized conditions in order to weaken the analyte-matrix interactions and increase the analyte-extractant interactions.

There is a continuous development of sample-treatment procedures for the isolation of pesticides in samples with relatively high fat content, such as olive oil and olives. The preparation of oil samples for their determination by chromatographic techniques requires the removal of the fatty components from the sample. The main problem associated when working with this kind of samples is that dirty extracts may harm the instruments employed. For this reason, proper extraction and clean-up steps are required. In addition, the different nature and physicochemical properties of the classes of pesticides to be analyzed makes it more complex to select the appropriate extraction methodology.

There are numerous extraction and clean-up procedures. However, the most common ones are solid-liquid or liquid-liquid extraction, gel permeation-chromatography (GPC) and solid-phase extraction (SPE) [6-8].

Solid-Liquid Extraction

In this case, the sample comes to contact with an appropriate solvent. After that, different procedures can be applied to homogenize both phases: ultrasonic agitation and microwave extraction.

Ultrasonic agitation: the solvent interacts with the sample simply by a shaking process. Ultrasonic radiation (frequency of 25-40 Hz) causes the vibration of the molecules, increasing the collision between them. Hence, the contact between sample and solvent is enhanced. After the analyte is dissolved in the extractant, a filtration step and the evaporation of the solvent are required.

Microwave extraction: samples are enclosed in high quality Teflon vessels together with the solvent and heated to a controlled temperature with microwave power, being the extract filtered when the process finishes. Electromagnetic irradiation is used to heat the solvent that acts as extractant, which is in most cases a mixture between hexane and acetone.

Liquid-Liquid Extraction

Usually, it has been the chosen method for the extraction, preconcentration and clean-up of liquid samples. It is based on the relative solubility of the analyte in two different immiscible liquids; therefore, it is an extraction of a substance from one liquid phase into another liquid phase. The liquid sample comes to contact with an appropriate solvent (immiscible with the sample) and, after a mixing time, both phases (sample and extractant) are separated. During the mixing period, the analyte is distributed between both phases until it reaches the equilibrium.

The $K_{O/W}$ value is critical to decide the appropriate extractant. If this value is high, it indicates that the analyte tends to dissolve in the organic phase instead of in water. As a general rule, the organic solvents selected are those one that present high affinity for the analytes, are immiscible with the sample and volatile (to evaporate them easily and preconcentrate the analytes).

Gel-Permeation Chromatography

It is probably the most extensively used technique for the analysis of pesticide residues in olive oil, usually after a liquid-liquid extraction. In this technique, an aliquot of an olive oil extract (obtained from the extraction step) is injected into the GPC system. The selected fraction is collected and, after a solvent-exchange step, the sample is analyzed by gas chromatography. A GPC system is composed of a chromatographic pump, a fraction collector and a detector. The columns are made from polymeric porous microspheres that enable the separation of compounds according to their molecular weights (which are related to the size of the compound). Using this principle, the pesticide fraction is separated from the triglyceride fraction, which presents higher molecular weight. In GPC, the compounds are eluted from higher to lower molecular weight.

Solid-Phase Extraction

It is a separation process by which compounds that are dissolved or suspended in a liquid mixture are separated from other compounds in the mixture according to their physical and chemical properties. SPE is used to concentrate and purify samples for analysis and to isolate the analytes of interest from a wide variety of matrices.

SPE uses the affinity of the analytes dissolved or suspended in a liquid (known as the mobile phase) for a solid through which the sample is passed (known as the stationary phase) to separate a mixture into desired and undesired components. The result is that either the desired analytes of interest or undesired impurities in the sample are retained on the stationary phase. The portion that passes through the stationary phase is collected or discarded, depending on whether it contains the desired analytes or undesired impurities. If the portion retained on the stationary phase includes the desired analytes, they can then be removed from the stationary phase for collection in an additional step, in which the stationary phase is rinsed with an appropriate eluent.

The stationary phase comes in the form of a packed syringe-shaped cartridge, each of which can be mounted on its specific type of extraction manifold. The manifold allows multiple samples to be processed by holding several SPE media in place and allowing for an equal number of samples to pass through them simultaneously. A typical cartridge SPE manifold can accommodate up to 24 cartridges and is equipped with a vacuum port. Application of vacuum speeds up the extraction process by pulling the liquid sample through the stationary phase. The analytes are collected in sample tubes inside or below the manifold after they pass through the stationary phase. Solid phase extraction cartridges are available with a variety of stationary phases, each of which can separate analytes according to different chemical properties. Most stationary phases are based on silica that has been bonded to a specific functional group. Gas chromatography (GC) is an analytical technique widely used for separating and analysing compounds that can be vaporized without decomposition [9,10]. Typical uses of GC include testing the purity of a particular substance, or separating the different components of a mixture. In GC, the mobile phase is a carrier gas, usually an inert gas such as helium or an unreactive gas such as nitrogen. The stationary phase is a microscopic layer of liquid or polymer on an inert solid support, inside a piece of glass or metal tubing called column. The instrument used to perform gas chromatography is called a gas chromatograph. A gas chromatograph uses a flow-through narrow tube known as the column, through which different chemical constituents of a sample pass in a gas stream (carrier gas, mobile phase) at different rates depending on their various chemical and physical properties and their interaction with a specific column filling, called the stationary phase. As the chemicals exit at the end of the column, they are detected and identified electronically. The function of the stationary phase in the column is to separate different components, causing each one to exit the column at a different time (retention time). Other parameters that can be used to alter the order or time of retention are the carrier gas flow rate, column length and the temperature.

In a GC analysis, a known volume of gaseous or liquid sample is injected into the head of the column using a microsyringe. As the carrier gas sweeps the analyte molecules through the column, this motion is inhibited by the adsorption of the analyte molecules either onto the column walls or onto packing materials in the column. The rate at which the molecules progress along the column depends on the strength of adsorption, which in turn depends on the type of molecule and on the stationary phase materials. Since each type of molecule has a different rate of progression, the various components of the mixture of analytes are separated as they progress along the column and reach the end of the column at different times. A detector is used to monitor the outlet stream from the column; thus, the time at which each component reaches the outlet and the amount of that component can be determined.

The column(s) in a GC are contained in an oven, the temperature of which is precisely controlled electronically. The rate at which a sample passes through the column is directly proportional to the temperature of the column. The higher the column temperature, the faster the sample moves through the column. However, the faster a sample moves through the column, the less it interacts with the stationary phase, and the less the analytes are separated. Two types of columns are used in GC:

- Packed columns are 1.5–10 m in length and have an internal diameter of 2–4 mm. The tubing is usually made of stainless steel or glass and contains a packing of finely divided, inert, solid support material (e.g. diatomaceous earth) that is coated with a liquid or solid stationary phase. The nature of the coating material determines what type of materials will be most strongly adsorbed.
- Capillary columns have a very small internal diameter, in the order of a few tenths of millimeters, and lengths between 25–60 meters are common. Most capillary columns are made of fused-silica with a polyimide outer coating. These columns are flexible, so a very long column can be wound into a small coil.

The most common detectors in GC until recent years were the flame ionization detector (FID), the thermal conductivity detector (TCD) and the electron capture detector (ECD). However, nowadays most of the developed analytical methods use a mass spectrometry (MS) detector. MS is an analytical technique that measures the mass-to-charge ratio of charged particles. It is used for determining masses of particles, for determining the elemental composition of a sample or molecule, and for elucidating the chemical structures of molecules.

7. Analysis of Pesticides in Olive Oil and Olives

On average, 5 kg of olives are required for the production of 1 L of oil. Taking into account that most pesticides are lipophilic, a concentration effect could occur when obtaining the olive oil. Thus, MRL for pesticides have been set by the European Union in both olives and olive oil. For this reason, our research group has developed analytical methods that allow the analysis of the selected plaguicides in olive oil [11] and olives [12]. For olive oil samples, the preparation procedure included a liquid-liquid extraction followed by GPC clean-up step. The detection of the pesticides was performed making use of GC coupled to mass spectrometry. The following Table shows the retention times (t_R) and analytical parameters obtained for each selected pesticide. DL and QL stand for detection and quantification limits. Figure 2 shows a chromatogram of these pesticides in an olive oil sample. It can be observed the total separation of the pesticides, being the number of the peaks the same ones assigned to the pesticides in Table 5. For olive samples, approximately 130 g of olives (including the seeds) were first crushed by means of a hammer mill. Afterwards, a 100 g portion was weighed in a glass tube and 50 g of anhydrous sodium sulphate were added. The sample was then extracted with an adequate organic solvent and a GPC-based clean-up procedure was applied to the fatty residue obtained after the extraction of the pesticides from the olives. Finally, their detection was performed by means of GC-MS. In a similar way to olive oil, the analytical parameters of the system for olives are shown in Table 6.

The procedures previously detailed were applied to the determination of the cited pesticides in olives and olive oil samples. In Table 7, the fourteen detected pesticides in real samples are shown. In particular, the herbicides diuron, terbuthylazine and endosulfan sulfate were found in many samples. Although other pesticides were also detected, in most cases the levels were below the QL of the system.

Influence of Harvesting Method

As it was commented in Section 3, there are different olive harvesting methods. Depending on this, the olive fruits can be grouped into three categories: a) fruits picked directly from the tree without any contact with the soil (flight olives); b) fruits picked from the ground (soil olives); and c) fruits that are not separated before the elaboration process (non-separated olives).

Table 5. Parameters of the GC-MS system for the selected pesticides in olive oil

No.	Plaguicide	t_R (min)	Linear Range (μg kg^{-1})	DL(μg kg^{-1})	QL(μg kg^{-1})
1	Diuron	6.908	5-1000	0.5	5
2	α-HCH	11.265	1-1000	0.5	1
3	Dimethoate	11.760	20-400	10	20
4	Simazine	11.971	3-2000	1	3
5	Atrazine	12.095	5-1000	2	5

6	Trietazine	12.621	10-800	5	10
7	β-HCH	12.644	0.5-1000	0.2	0.5
8	Terbuthylazine	12.666	1-1000	0.5	1
9	δ-HCH	12.750	1-1000	0.5	1
10	Diazinon	12.801	5-1000	2	5
11	Lindane	14.500	0.5-1000	0.2	0.5
12	Formothion	14.916	20-1000	10	20
13	Chlorpyrifos-methyl	15.849	5-2000	1	5
14	Heptachlor	16.861	3-1000	1	3
15	Carbaryl	17.110	5-2000	1	5
16	Pirimifos-methyl	17.833	1-2000	0.5	1
17	Terbutrine	18.125	20-1000	5	20
18	Fenitrothion	18.165	3-2000	1	3
19	Chlorpyrifos	19.208	0.5-1500	0.2	0.5
20	Aldrin	19.386	10-1000	5	10
21	Heptachlor-epox-a	21.736	5-2000	1	5
22	Heptachlor-epox-b	21.990	5-2000	1	5
23	Folpet	22.882	10-2000	5	10
24	α-Endosulfan	23.931	5-2000	1	5
25	Dieldrin	25.475	5-2000	1	5
26	Endrin	26.633	10-2000	5	10
27	β-Endosulfan	27.327	5-2000	1	5
28	DDD	27.767	0.5-2000	0.2	0.5
29	Endosulfan sulfate	29.393	5-1000	2	5
30	DDT	29.908	5-2000	1	5
31	Triphenylphosphate	30.63	Recovery standard		

The separation of flight and soil olive fruits before olive oil elaboration is critical in order to obtain appropriate results (high-quality virgin olive oil). If both fruits are not separated, the quality of the oil and the percentage of extra virgin olive oil obtained diminish. In addition, the harvesting method may be very important for the presence of pesticide residues in olives, especially herbicides that are applied to the soil.

Data from Table 7 show that herbicide diuron was quantified in a high number of samples in soil olives and olive oil. In four of them, the levels were higher than the MRL established by the European Union (0.2 and 0.8 mg kg^{-1}, respectively). Terbuthylazine and endosulfan sulfate were also quantified in many samples with values over the MRL in some of them, being the established MRLs 0.05 and 0.2 mg kg^{-1} for both pesticides in olives and olive oil, respectively.

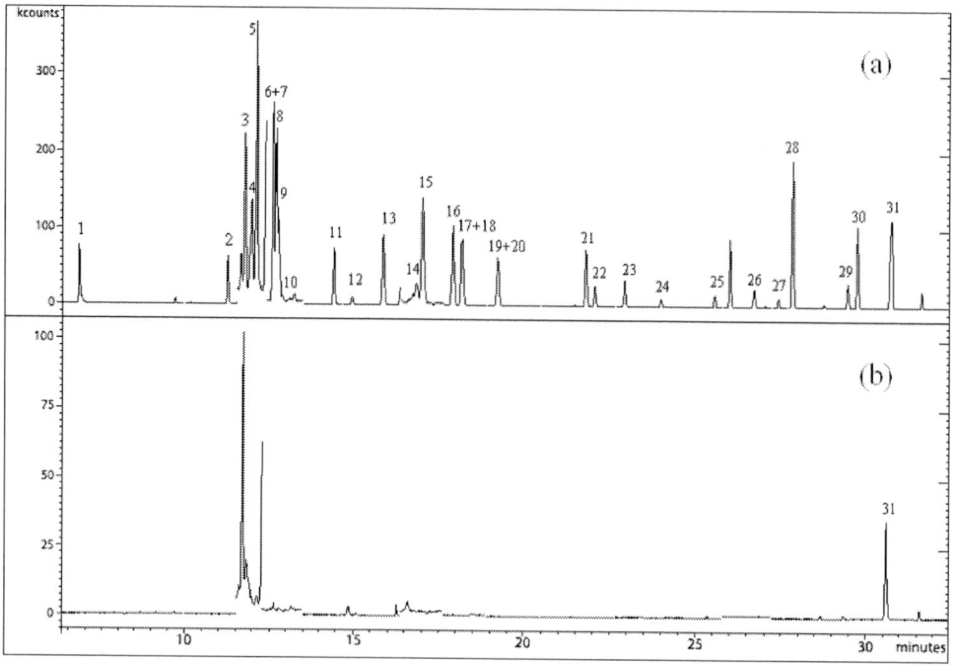

Figure 2. GC-MS chromatogram corresponding to: (a) standard of pesticides in olive oil; (b) olive oil without pesticides added.

These results suggest that herbicide residues are mainly caused by the contamination of the olives when they come to contact with the soil after falling down [11,13]. The levels of herbicides found in soil olives have been significantly higher than those ones found in flight olives, which have not been in contact with the soil. However, the levels of endosulfan sulfate are very similar in soil and flight olives.

The reason is that this pesticide is applied by spray in the atmosphere, and not on the soil. Hence, it can be carried large distances through the air and the most plausible way of contamination is when the olives are still on the tree. This mechanism of contamination would explain some cases when this pesticide has been detected in olives even when it has not been directly applied to the tree. In one olive mill, where the fruits are not separated before the olive oil elaboration, low levels of pesticides were observed, finding only one sample with terbuthylazine levels higher than its MRL.

Influence of Washing in Olive Mill

Taking into account the few bibliographic data about the fate of the pesticides after their application on the olive groves, it would be interesting to evaluate what fraction of the pesticides could be eliminated from the olives after the washing process in the olive mill, previous selection of a group of pesticides which frequently appears in these samples. The selected plaguicides were diuron, terbuthylazine and endosulfan sulfate.

Table 6. Parameters of the GC-MS system for the selected pesticides in olives

No.	Plaguicide	t_R (min)	Linear Range (μg kg^{-1})	DL (μg kg^{-1})	QL (μg kg^{-1})
1	Diuron	6.908	1.25-250	0.12	1.25
2	α-HCH	11.265	0.25-250	0.12	0.25
3	Dimethoate	11.760	5-100	2.50	5
4	Simazine	11.971	0.75-125	0.25	0.75
5	Atrazine	12.095	1.25-250	0.5	1.25
6	Trietazine	12.621	2.50-200	1.25	2.5
7	β-HCH	12.644	0.12-250	0.05	0.12
8	Terbuthylazine	12.666	0.25-250	0.12	0.25
9	δ-HCH	12.750	0.25-250	0.12	0.25
10	Diazinon	12.801	1.25-250	0.5	1.25
11	Lindane	14.500	0.12-250	0.05	0.12
12	Formothion	14.916	5-250	2.5	5
13	Chlorpyrifos-methyl	15.849	1.25-500	0.25	1.25
No.	Plaguicide	t_R (min)	Linear Range (μg kg^{-1})	DL (μg kg^{-1})	QL (μg kg^{-1})
14	Heptachlor	16.861	0.75-250	0.25	0.75
15	Carbaryl	17.110	1.25-500	0.25	1.25
16	Pirimifos-methyl	17.833	0.25-500	0.12	0.25
17	Terbutrine	18.125	5-250	1.25	5
18	Fenitrothion	18.165	0.75-500	0.25	0.75
19	Chlorpyrifos	19.208	0.12-375	0.05	0.12
20	Aldrin	19.386	2.5-250	1.25	2.5
21	Heptachlor-epox-a	21.736	1.25-500	0.25	1.25
22	Heptachlor-epox-b	21.990	1.25-500	0.25	1.25
23	Folpet	22.882	10-2000	5	10
24	α-Endosulfan	23.931	5-2000	1	5
25	Dieldrin	25.475	5-2000	1	5
26	Oxyfluorfen	25.918	2.5-250	1.25	2.5
27	Endrin	26.633	10-2000	5	10
28	β-Endosulfan	27.327	5-2000	1	5
29	DDD	27.767	0.5-2000	0.2	0.5
30	Endosulfan sulfate	29.393	5-1000	2	5
31	DDT	29.908	5-2000	1	5

The fruit goes into the olive-oil mill with a great quantity of impurities, leaves, branches, mud, etc, which are necessary to eliminate. Therefore, for this purpose, cleaners and washing devices are employed to eliminate impurities (Section 3), especially present in soil olives. Some olive mills separate flight and soil olives, whereas others treat all the fruits together, without any separation process.

Table 7. Number of samples with pesticides in olive and olive oil samples

Plaguicide	Olives			Olive oil		
	Soil	Flight	Non-separated	Soil	Flight	Non-separated
	n=50	n=20	n=24	n=15	n=10	n=8
Diuron	46	13	20	15	10	6
α-HCH	6	2	4	0	0	1
Simazine	2	1	1	5	2	2
Dimethoate	2	0	0	0	0	0
Atrazine	5	0	1	0	0	0
β-HCH	6	2	1	0	0	0
Terbuthylazine	42	13	24	15	10	7
Lindane	2	1	2	0	0	0
Carbaryl	2	1	3	0	0	0
Chlorpyrifos	2	0	0	5	2	2
α-Endosulfan	7	10	2	2	2	0
Dieldrin	2	0	0	0	0	0
β-Endosulfan	2	0	0	0	0	0
Endosulfan sulfato	26	9	16	9	9	5

n = total number of samples analyzed.

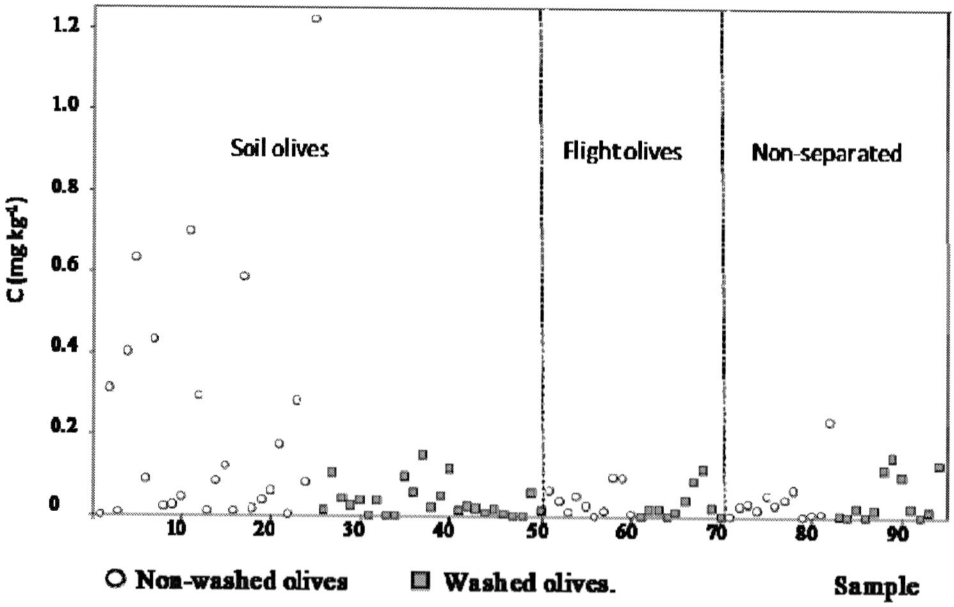

Figure 3. Concentration of pesticides in washed and non-washed olives.

Our research group presented the first exhaustive study of the influence of the olives washing in the mills over the concentration of pesticides[14-16]. The obtained results in flight, soil and non-separated olives after the washing process are shown in Figure 3, where the total concentration of the three selected pesticides is represented for 47 samples (non-washed and washed olives). The most outstanding conclusion is the reduction in the levels of plaguicides in soil olives after the washing process when compared to the same olive samples before the washing step. Only two samples presented levels higher than the legislated MRL for the herbicide terbuthylazine. It can be observed that the washing process significantly diminishes the levels of residues of plaguicides in soil olives, while the influence of the washing step is not clearly appreciated in flight olives. In the case of non-separated olives, it is interesting to remark that some of the washed olives present higher levels of pesticides than the non-washed ones. This can be due to the contamination of pesticides-free olives during the washing process. The washing machines for the olives are cleaned and filled with fresh water at the starting of the day. With this water, up to 160000 kg of olives can be washed before the water is changed next day. The water can be contaminated after the washing of soil olives, therefore contaminating following pesticides-free olives in the washing process. The washing waters (before and after the washing process) from the the olive mill were analyzed and the obtained results confirmed this theory [16].

Conclusions

The production of virgin olive oil has increased in recent years and it is being exported to different countries, representing an important part of the economy in some Mediterranean countries. As we described in the first part of this chapter, it poses a lot of beneficial properties for the human health. However, it is important to carry out exhaustive quality controls in order to maintain its high standards. One of the most important ones is the analysis of residues of pesticides, which can be very dangerous for the human body, presenting different adverse effects over the organism depending on their toxicity.

Here, we have described the most common procedures developed for the analysis of pesticides in olives and olive oil. It has been shown that some pesticides are commonly found in these samples, although usually at levels below the established MRLs. In addition, the separation of flight and soil olives, together with the washing process in the mills, is a critical step in order to control the levels of herbicides. Hence, the exhaustive analyses that are routinely carried out for pesticides should be kept in order to continue ensuring the safety of the virgin olive oil.

References

[1] El, S.N., and Karakaya, S. (2009). Olive tree (Olea europaea) leaves: Potential beneficial effects on human health. *Nutrition Reviews*, 67, 632-638.

[2] Cicerale, S., Lucas, L., and Keast, R. (2010). Biological activities of phenolic compounds present in virgin olive oil. *International Journal of Molecular Sciences*, 11, 458-479.

[3] International Olive Council (2010). *Trade Standard Applying to Olive Oils and Olive-Pomace Oils. COI/T.15/NC.*

[4] LeDoux, M. (2011). Analytical methods applied to the determination of pesticide residues in foods of animal origin. A review of the past two decades. *Journal of Chromatography A*, 1218, 1021-1036.

[5] Tankiewicz, M., Fenik, J., and Biziuk, M. (2010). Determination of organophosphorus and organonitrogen pesticides in water samples. *TrAC Trends in Analytical Chemistry*, 29, 1050-1063.

[6] Gilbert-López, B., García-Reyes, J.F., and Molina-Díaz, A. (2009). Sample treatment and determination of pesticide residues in fatty vegetable matrices: A review. *Talanta*, 79, 109-128.

[7] Mukherjee, I., and Gopal, M. (1996). Chromatographic techniques in the analysis of organochlorine pesticide residues. *Journal of Chromatography A*, 754, 33-42.

[8] Walters, S.M. (1990). Clean-up techniques for pesticides in fatty foods. *Analytica Chimica Acta*, 236, 77-82.

[9] Harris, D.C. (2007). *Quantitative Chemical Analysis*. Freeman and Company, New York.

[10] Skoog, D.A., West, D.M., and Holler, F.J. (1996). *Fundamentals of Analytical Chemistry*. Saunders College, Philadelphia.

[11] Guardia-Rubio, M., Fernández-de Córdova, M.L., Ayora-Cañada, M.J., and Ruiz-Medina, A. (2006). Simplified pesticide multiresidue analysis in virgin olive oil by gas chromatography with thermoionic specific, electron-capture and mass spectrometric detection. *Journal of Chromatography A*, 1108, 231-239.

[12] Guardia-Rubio, M., Marchal-López, R.M., Ayora-Cañada, M.J., and Ruiz-Medina, A. (2007). Determination of pesticides in olives by gas chromatography using different detection systems. *Journal of Chromatography A*, 1145, 195-203.

[13] Guardia-Rubio, M., Ruiz-Medina, A., Molina-Díaz, A., and Ayora-Cañada, M.J. (2006). Influence of harvesting method and washing on the presence of pesticide residues in olives and olive oil. *Journal of Agricultural and Food Chemistry*, 54, 8538-8544.

[14] Guardia Rubio, M., Ruiz Medina, A., Pascual Reguera, M.I., and Fernández de Córdova, M.L. (2007). Multiresidue analysis of three groups of pesticides in washing waters from olive processing by solid-phase extraction-gas chromatography with electron capture and thermionic specific detection. *Microchemical Journal*, 85, 257-264.

[15] Guardia-Rubio, M., Ayora-Cañada, M.J., and Ruiz-Medina, A. (2007). Effect of washing on pesticide residues in olives. *Journal of Food Science*, 72, C139-C143.

[16] Guardia-Rubio, M., Ruiz-Medina, A., Molina-Díaz, A., and Ayora-Cañada, M.J. (2008). Pesticide residues in washing water of olive oil mills: Effect on olive washing efficiency and decontamination proposal. *Journal of the Science of Food and Agriculture*, 88, 2467-2473.

In: Vegetable Consumption and Health: New Research
Editors: Claudia Wilson and Melinda Morree
ISBN: 978-1-62100-941-2

Chapter 3

Human Photosynthesis

Arturo Solís-Herrera*, María del Carmen Arias Esparza, Ruth Isabel Solís-Arias, Paola Eugenia Solís-Arias and Martha Patricia Solís-Arias

Human Photosynthesis Study Center. Av. Aguascalientes Norte 607, Pulgas Pandas Sur, CP 20230, Aguascalientes, México

Abstract

The advent of photosynthesis is one of the central events in the early development of life on Earth. The origin and evolution of photosynthesis, however, has long remained unresolved. Any studious individual who wishes to appreciate the big picture of how photosynthesis works and how it fits into the broad scope of scientific inquiry needs to have at least a rudimentary understanding of numerous fields of science. This is an increasingly difficult task in this age of scientific specialization, because no one can truly be an expert in all areas. The intent of this paper is not to advance knowledge on the plant process presently called photosynthesis, a very important photochemical process considered to be the origin of the food chain that is still not yet completely understood in spite of the fact it has already seen 350 years of study. Rather, this article attempts to provide a starting point for an unsuspected metabolic pathway over and above what we know about plants, the hitherto unknown capability of Melanin, the animal analogue to Chlorophyll, to harvest electromagnetic radiations to use as energy to dissociate the water molecule with a subsequent release of energy. An analogue process with that of plants, so similar in animal cells to the first step in plant photosynthesis (absorption of light/dissociation of water), that we have named it "Human Photosynthesis."

* Phone: +52 449 153 2790, +52 449 912 1358, +52 449 912 1374. comagua2000@yahoo.com.

INTRODUCTION

Photosynthesis According to Textbooks

The term photosynthesis literally means building up, putting together, or assembly by light. As commonly used, photosynthesis describes the process by which plants synthesize organic compounds from inorganic raw materials in the presence of sunlight. That is, plants tap sunlight energy to make sugars out of carbon dioxide gas and water. The sugars, when combined with the minerals from the soil, are used as building materials to make plant tissue, proteins, fats, and all other chemicals needed for life. All forms of life in this universe require energy and building blocks for growth and maintenance. It is well known that algae, higher plants, and certain types of bacteria also capture energy directly from solar radiation and utilize it for the synthesis of essential food materials. Nevertheless, textbooks continue, up to now, to erroneously perpetuate the concept that animals cannot use sunlight directly as source of energy, thus they must obtain their energy and building materials from the plants they eat or from eating other animals that have eaten plants. This thinking, despite its errors, recognizes that the ultimate source of all metabolic energy in our planet is the sun.

Sunlight is pure energy, and photosynthesis is essential for maintaining all forms of life on earth. If we think that plant photosynthesis is the most important biological process, then the substance that makes plants look green, chlorophyll, should be considered to be the most important biological molecule so long as we continue to think that animal life appeared later in this planet. Photosynthesis could thus be regarded as the process by which radiant energy from the sun is converted into chemical energy for plant tissue.

All plants and animals carry out the process of respiration (in mitochondria), whereby O_2 is taken from the atmosphere by living tissue to be converted into carbohydrates and other tissue constituents and eventually to CO_2 and H_2O, with the simultaneous liberation of energy. This energy is stored in adenosine triphosphate (ATP) and is utilized for the normal functioning of the organism. However, ATP cannot be considered as energy stored, because every ATP molecule must be reconstituted every 20 seconds on the average. Respiration thus causes a decrease in the organic matter and O_2 content, and an increase in the CO_2 content of the planet [1].

All forms of life on earth then depend on the energy that comes from the sun. And yet, it is essential for this photonic energy to be transformed into a different kind of energy, which might in turn be used to impel a second reaction and then a third one and so on, until finally a chemical self-sustainable system would emerge that could eventually go into Darwinian evolution. Observing nature carefully, we know that Photonic Energy must first be transduced into Chemical Energy. Living things containing chlorophyll are thought to be the oldest organisms because they take advantage of the transduction performed by the well-known, and poorly understood, water-splitting capability of chlorophyll. However, in order to transduce photonic energy into chemical energy, chlorophyll needs to be inside a living thing, e.g., a living cell. Otherwise, the chlorophyll molecule loses this capability in less than twenty seconds. This fact should make scientists think that life must have come first and chlorophyll second. Published data by several researchers has shown that phylogenetic analysis of small-subunit rRNA suggests that green nonsulfur bacteria are the earliest evolving photosynthetic lineage [2]. On the one hand, Gupta et al. [3] concluded that heliobacteria are the earliest evolving photosynthetic lineage and that this lineage subsequently diverged to green nonsulfur bacteria, cyanobacteria, green sulfur bacteria, and purple bacteria, in that order. The conflicting trees derived from such studies indicate that extrapolating the evolution of photosynthesis from non-photosynthesis gene trees may be invalid. Therefore, that road seems to be a dead-end.

On the other hand, the very first spark of life had to happen in a completely sterile environment, i.e., with no other form of life present; otherwise it could have been instantly absorbed or devoured. Therefore, the question remains, where did the chemical energy needed for the first spark of life come from? Discussing photosynthesis is not an easy task because of the span of the time scale involved that goes from the cosmic to the unimaginably fast, i.e., from the origin of the Earth 4.5 billion years ago, to molecular processes that take less than a picosecond, a range of nearly thirty orders of magnitude [4].

Knowledge regarding the photosynthesis process in plants has gradually increased; however, the process is not yet completely understood. Nevertheless, plant photosynthesis is not only a very well-accepted biochemical process, it is also considered to be the basis for the origin of life. Given the significance of the transduction of photonic energy into chemical energy, and due to the belief that plants are unique in this regard, the plant kingdom is considered to be the basis of the food chain with two coupled "sub-cycles" between food producers (plants), and food consumers (animals).

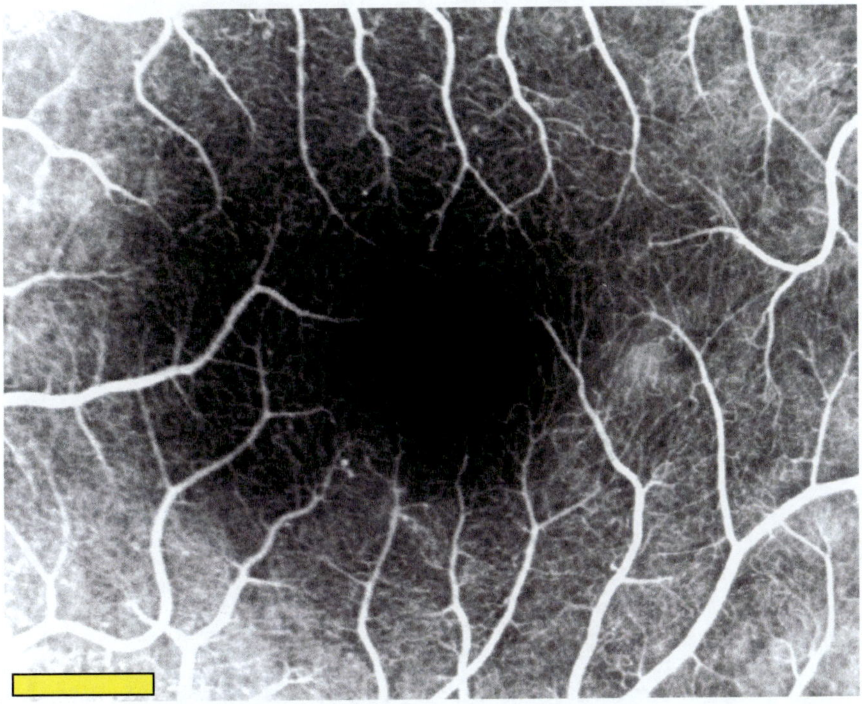

Figure 1. Vascular distribution of the human macular zone *in vivo,* the region of highest visual acuity. The dark coloration of the central nonvascular zone is due to the presence of melanin behind the retinal tissue. Calibration bar 200 microns.

Melanin Is the Answer

In 1990, we began a study looking for new treatments for the three main causes of blindness. The main variable in our study was the general characteristics of the blood vessels in the optic nerve and retina. Our hypotheses was based on the fact, firm at that time, that if glucose was the universal currency of energy for all tissue blood vessels must, therefore, be the only source of nutrients for the retina and optic nerve. Thus, we were looking for early anomalies in the size, diameter, and/or changes in the wall of blood vessels so we could modulate these changes early using mainly pharmacological agents, in order to diminish the anatomical alterations that eventually would cause vision loss. Our equipment was modified according to our theory so we could get the highest possible magnification that would facilitate finding the earliest anatomical and functional alterations in the blood vessels.

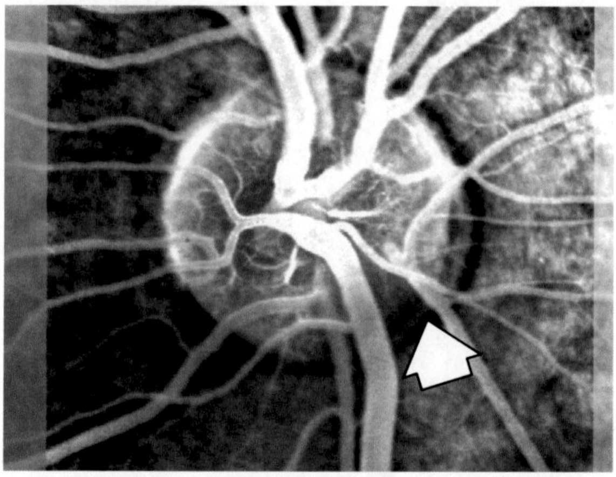

Figure 2. Capillarity of the Optic Nerve *in vivo*. The magnification reached allowed us to see the finest details. Unexpectedly, we could also see the melanin much better (arrow head) forming a rim around the optic disc.

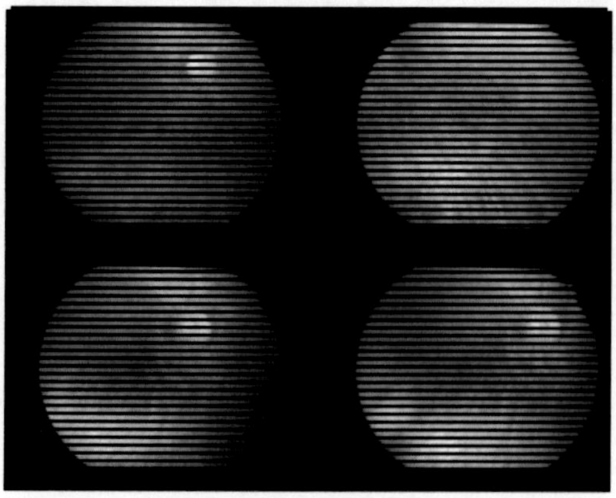

Figure 3. Choroidal blood vessels. Photography of the ocular fundus *in vivo* taken with a wavelength of 800 nm. This type of electromagnetic radiation produces a surprisingly clear image of the choroid, a layer of tissue subjacent to the retina. Blood vessels are observed like white strings intertwined with a dark color substance, Melanin.

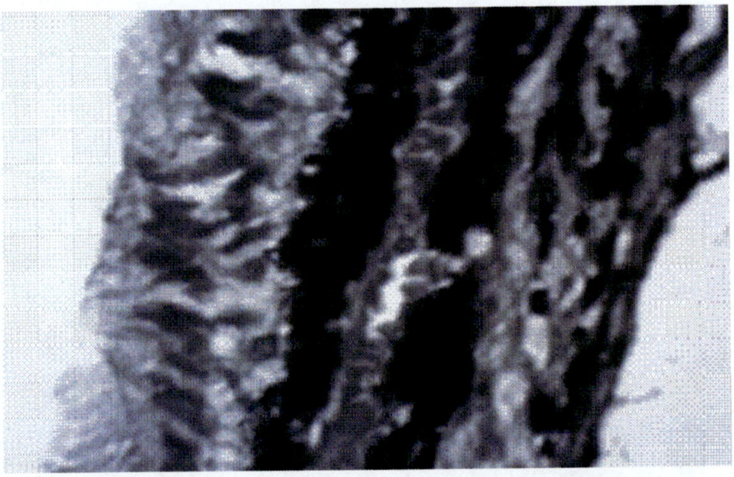

Figure 4. Microphotography of the Choroid. Histological aspect of Melanin situated between the different layers of blood vessels normally present in this tissue. H and E, 40 X. Solís-Herrera.

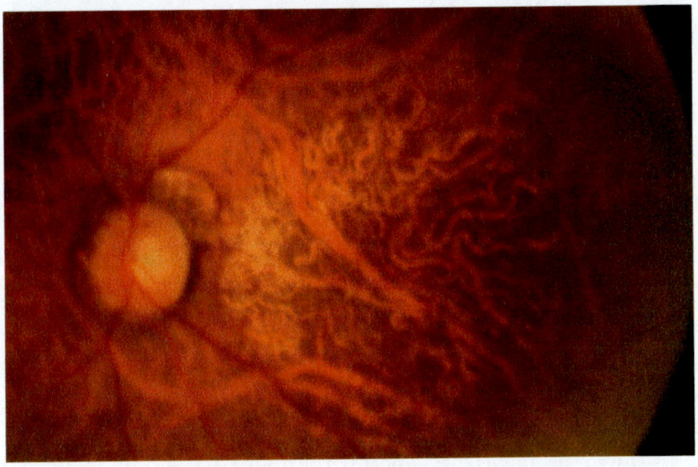

Figure 5. The Choroid observed *in vivo* with polychromatic (white) light. The resolution is less than with monochromatic light. In spite of that, we could still see the ever-present melanin around the optic disc intertwined with the choroidal blood vessels.

Our findings in human retina break the paradigm that the capability to harvest photonic energy, and its ulterior transduction into chemical energy, is an exclusive characteristic of the photosystem of plants, constituted in order of abundance in nature by Light/Water/ Chlorophyll. Human beings also have an equivalent photosystem, constituted by Light/Melanin/Water in order of their abundance in nature. In other words, our own body can effectuate the process of water dissociation, similar to the first step that occurs in plants; in both cases, there is separation of the water molecule, a vital part of any process in cellular physiology. Astonishingly, the main product of this reaction is diatomic hydrogen, and not oxygen, because hydrogen is the energy carrier by excellence in the whole universe. On the other hand, oxygen is toxic at any level.

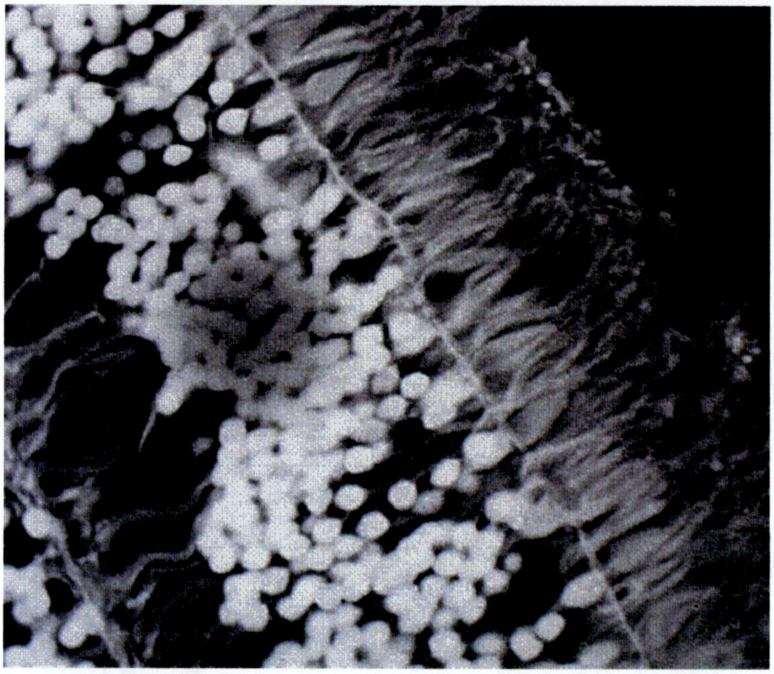

Figure 6. The most energy-demanding layer of the eye, and probably of the human body, is the Photoreceptor layer (Solís-Herrera, 2002). Strikingly, there are no blood vessels at all. However, the energy requirements are ten times those of the cerebral cortex, six times those of the coronary arteries, and three times those of the renal cortex.

The principles of human photosynthesis could explain why human beings with higher levels of water dissociation capability have cells with a lower number of mitochondria, up to 83% less. Other interesting examples to consider in humans are hemoglobin and erythrocytes, because they are the only cells in the human body that normally do not have mitochondria, and if they don't have mitochondria, where is their energy coming from? Erythrocytes absorb wavelengths close to 400 nm, and, therefore, they reflect wavelengths of 700nm, that is why we see them red. Thus, the necessary energy for their metabolic requirements could come from the blue zone of the electromagnetic spectrum.

In oxygenic photosynthesis, water is split at a Mn4Ca complex bound to the proteins of the photosystem II (PSII). Powered by four quanta of visible light, four electrons and four protons are removed from two water molecules before di-oxygen is released [5]. This is the main analogy with human photosynthesis. In plant photosynthesis, green plants use the energy of sunlight to convert carbon dioxide into hydrocarbons that promote plant growth while generating oxygen from water and releasing oxygen to the atmosphere. All animals, including humans, depend either directly or indirectly on this source of food and oxygen. Consequently, photosynthesis is considered to be the most important chemical process on Earth [6].

Thus, all life on Earth depends on photosynthesis for food and oxygen. The origin of this crucial process in green plants is a longstanding problem in biology, and a number of different theories have been proposed to explain it. But there has been no clear evidence to support any of these proposed theories.

C3 and C4 Plants

Sour grasses are C4 species, while sweet grasses are C3 species, with a geographical separation of warm season "sour" grasses from cool season "sweet" grasses that has long been noticed by pastoralists. During his research life, J.C. Bose carried out important and thought-provoking experiments on photosynthesis. In the simplest terms, Dr. Bose described photosynthesis in plants as the process by which CO_2 and H_2O are taken up, forming carbohydrate and releasing oxygen, using light. During his research, Dr. Bose made one of the most fascinating instruments: The Photosynthesis Recorder, which can detect the formation of carbohydrate as a millionth of a gram per minute and record the rate of photosynthetic activity.

Sir J.C. Bose observed that "while the juice of the plant was practically neutral in winter and spring, it was very strongly acid in summer." Furthermore, "the acidity of the plants was found to be due to the presence of malic and oxalic acids, the latter in small quantities." It is quite astonishing that as early as 1924, Bose had visualized the idea of operation, in Hydrilla, of a quite different photosynthetic pathway, which utilizes malate [7].

The primary route of carbon assimilation through Calvin-Benson-Bassham cycle, or C3-pathway, was established by the research group of Melvin Calvin, Andy Benson and their coworkers. The variant of carbon assimilation is Crassulacean Acid metabolism (CAM), which also uses malate and other acids to concentrate CO_2 inside the cells during darkness (or night); these acids are used up during subsequent daytime.

Bose said: "The organic acids stored during the night (in succulent plants) provide indirect material for photosynthesis during the day in the form of CO_2. The *Hydrilla* plant appeared to be the most suitable for further investigation on the subject that the organic acid served directly for photosynthesis." J.C. Bose examined the effects of several compounds, which either stimulated or inhibited the rate of photosynthesis depending on the nature and concentration of the compounds. His observations on the stimulatory effects by almost infinitesimal quantities of different chemical agents were triggered by a casual observation that the rate of photosynthesis in certain water plants increased sharply during a thunderstorm. Bose attributed this phenomenon to the oxides of nitrogen produced by electric discharges in the atmosphere. He found that the photosynthesis of *Hydrilla verticillata* was tripled by nitric acid and doubled by thyroid gland extract. Iodine and formaldehyde increased the photosynthetic rate 60% and 80%, respectively. In maize, a C4 plant, exposure to light initiates the bundle sheath-specific expression of Rubisco. The basal energy required per CO_2 assimilation in C4 photosynthesis is the sum of energy to support the C4 and C3 cycles. 5 ATP, 2 NADPH required per CO_2 assimilated (2 ATP for the C4 cycle, 3 ATP, 2 NADPH for the C3 cycle). This, combined with the presence of stomata on the stems, starch in stem chlorenchyma, and light-dependent fixation of atmospheric CO_2 by the stems, suggests they contribute to carbon assimilation. The stems of Borszczowia have C3 type chlorenchyma cells scattered throughout the cortical tissue. They likely function to refix respired CO_2 in stems, since light-dependent fixation of external CO_2 is only observed under high atmospheric levels [8].

C4 photosynthesis, in its several forms, is essentially a biochemical CO_2 concentrating mechanism that increases the substrate CO_2 in the vicinity of ribulose bisphosphate carboxylase- oxygenase to overcome the competitive inhibition by O_2 and oxygenase activity of this enzyme [9].

It has long been recognized that photosynthesis in dense aquatic vegetation, whether composed of cyanobacteria, phytoplankton, seaweed, seagrass, or freshwater plants, can drive the pH of the water as high as 10, deplete the free CO_2 and even HCO_3 - to near zero, and produce O_2 that is double the air-equilibrium value [10]. Even under high atmospheric CO_2, such conditions likely occurred in the water on the early earth, as water bodies are rarely in equilibrium with air. However, they do not appear to possess C4 photosynthesis. It has been estimated that some 50% of submersed angiosperms have the capacity to use HCO_3 - actively in photosynthesis [11]. This facility is facultative and when upregulated, it probably can function in some species as a CCM [12]. Thus, when C4 photosynthesis is absent, the change from high to lower G values may be due to acclimation in some form(s) of HCO_3- use at low CO_2. In this regard, the dissolved CO_2 appears to be the effective agent resulting in up-regulation of HCO_3- use, more so than HCO_3- in the water [13]. However, upregulation of HCO_3- use is not the complete answer, as some species, including mosses, appear only able to use CO_2.

The notion that the aquatic environment is relatively "benign" for plants and lacks the selection pressure that resulted in terrestrial C4 CCMs is invalid. Aridity may not be a primary factor [14], but it is not uncommon to find freshwater systems and marine rock pools that are very unfavorable for C3 photosynthesis, with high daytime O_2, temperature, pH, and irradiance, and minimal inorganic carbon [15]. The situation is exacerbated by slow dissolution and diffusion of CO_2 in water, which has a diffusion resistance 10^4 times greater than air. These conditions rival any terrestrial extremes, and stress submersed photoautotrophs. It is not unreasonable to conclude that similar environments existed in the past, even when atmospheric CO_2 was high, because water and air are rarely in equilibrium in regards to CO_2 and O_2.

A plant or alga with the ability to minimize photorespiration, or offset CO_2 loss by taking it up at night in a CAM-like mode, would have an advantage in environments where CO_2 availability during the day can be severely limiting. HCO_3-, which in most fresh and marine waters is many-fold higher in concentration than dissolved CO_2. HCO_3-, use requires the organism to have a mechanism that can utilize this ion in photosynthesis, either by direct uptake through active transport or by its conversion in the boundary layer to CO_2 in an ATP-dependent acidification process.

In rough accordance with earlier estimates, recent in vivo 13C labeling experiments indicate that photorespiration is about 17% of photosynthesis for a well-watered and fertilized plant under temperate conditions [16]. And what is the biological function of the photorespiratory processes? In essence, it is quite simple—the synthesis of 2PG by RubP oxygenase as the primary reaction of the C2 cycle appears to have no "function" at all. However, in nature, closed roads like this in the metabolic pathways are virtually nonexistent. This concept is similar in regards to the function of melanin. Until now, the main reluctance to accept melanin as a molecule with biological activity has been its apparent stability.

LIGNIN, A KIND OF MELANIN?

Lignin, a plant constituent, is the second most abundant biopolymer on earth [17], and just like melanin, it is a conducting polymer; both are derivatives of the same aminoacid. Lignin is a polymer of aromatic subunits usually derived from phenylalanine. It serves as a matrix around the polysaccharide components of some plant cell walls, providing additional rigidity and compressive strength as well as rendering the walls hydrophobic and water impermeable. Terrestrial vascular plants may, therefore, have appeared only after the evolution of lignin biosynthesis, because structural support and water transport functions are central to the biology of higher land plants [18].

Trees have extreme needs for both structural support and water transport, processes both with significant energy requirements. Accordingly, they synthesize high levels of lignin in wood: 15 to 36% of the dry weight of wood is lignin [19]. Lignin is, therefore, one of the world's most abundant natural polymers, along with cellulose and chitin.

Lignin deposition can be induced in many cell types by disease or wounding, indicating that the genes involved in lignin biosynthesis respond to both developmental and environmental signals. Melanin deposition can also be induced in many cells types, by disease or wounding.

Phenylpropanoid compounds are so named because of the basic structure of a three-carbon side chain on an aromatic ring, which is derived from L-phenylalanine. Despite 50 years of investigation, the exact mechanisms and enzymology of lignin polymerization remain in doubt. A lot of mystery surrounds lignin as it also happens in regards to melanin.

Enough support exists, however, for the concept that lignin polymerization is not random but organized [20, 21, 22], and it is the same for melanin. Terashima [23] has argued convincingly that the lignin polymer formed in cell wall biosynthesis is a structurally ordered macromolecule formed by a regulated process. In regards to melanin, it is the same case, just in mice there are 100 genes controlling melanin expression.

A related question concerns the cellular origin of the lignin precursors and the time of lignin deposition. The work of Terashima and co-workers argues for regulated deposition during cell wall biosynthesis because of specific changes in composition that are found in the cell wall layers. Paradoxically, it appears that lignin deposition can occur in cells that are no longer alive [24], a process that might require transport from nearby cells still producing monolignols, perhaps ray parenchymal cells. A similar process happens in the skin with the translation of melanin from dermal melanocytes to the epidermal cells.

The complexity of the lignin structure has made analysis of polymerization mechanisms a challenging topic. It has been difficult to demonstrate that lignin structure deviates significantly from a random polymer; increasing evidence now suggests that monomer residues are organized within the lignin polymer, and research is focusing on the mechanisms that give rise to order. We can expect to understand, within the next decade, facets of the structure and biosynthesis of this complex polymer that have eluded explanation for the past 100 years. We could easily exchange the word "lignin" for the word "melanin" and find that the same is true for melanin.

Lignin is a major cell wall component in woody plants and grasses, comprising 15 to 25% of the plant's cell wall material. Structurally, lignin consists of a variety of phenylpropane monomeric units randomly coupled together by an assortment of carbon-carbon and ether linkages. In its native state in the cell wall, lignin probably exists as a three-dimensional polymeric network of essentially infinite mol wt, owing in part to its random origin from enzyme-initiated free radical polymerization reactions [25].

Lignin plays a crucial role in conducting water in plant stems. The polysaccharide components of plant cell walls are highly hydrophilic and thus permeable to water, whereas lignin is more hydrophobic. The cross-linking of polysaccharides by lignin is an obstacle for water absorption to the cell wall. Thus, lignin makes it possible for the plant's vascular tissue to conduct water efficiently; however we must think that this process (conducting water efficiently) requires energy. Cinnamaldehyde occurs widely, and closely related compounds give rise to lignin. All such compounds are biosynthesized starting from phenylalanine, like melanin itself, which undergoes conversion to cinnamoyl ester of coenzyme A.

At the moment, it is not possible to remove lignin from wood without at least partially degrading its polymeric network superstructure, like melanin, which cannot be removed from tissue in a pure form. As a result, practically all of the chemical and spectroscopic information about lignin has been obtained from lignin fragments isolated from lignocellulosics by chemical or mechanical treatments, sounding identical to the technical problems that present themselves with melanin. Lignin fragments obtained by these methods are typically polydisperse with regard to mol wt, are soluble in neutral organic solvents, are modified chemically, and lack many of the physical and mechanical properties associated with lignin *in situ.* If instead of "lignin" we write "melanin," the same is applicable.

Prolonged ethanol extraction of wood from a variety of softwood and hardwood species yields a low molecular wt (<2000) soluble lignin fraction that exhibits a strong UV absorption band at about 280 nm. However, this fraction, which accounts for only 3% of the lignin present in the wood, may not be representative of the bulk of the lignin in situ. Therefore, there are no suitable models that allow the study of lignin in situ—a striking coincidence to what happens with melanin.

Because of lignin's very high mol wt, interlocking three-dimensional network superstructure, and close physical and chemical association with polysaccharides, its properties and functions in the cell wall can be determined only from studies *in situ.* Complicated spectral effects occur in completely conjugated systems, thus it does not seem unreasonable to suppose that such a situation may exist within the high mol wt, rigid, three-dimensional lignin network found in situ and indeed in melanin, too.

Melanin and lignin are compounds that are very similar and important, functionally and from the structural point of view as well. Both compounds seem to be very stable; therefore they appear as biologically inactive. Melanin is an obligated component of the eye, and our finding of its capacity to split water and therefore produce energy explains very well several metabolic pathways in retina. On the other hand, lignin is an obligated component of the stem in plants, and the mystery about how plant sap is transported along the entire stem could be solved if we think of the possibility that lignin could produce energy by means of water dissociation, as melanin does.

During an investigation into seed vigor in cowpea, it was found that both the extent of water uptake and the rate of germination, especially after accelerated ageing, could be related to the color of the seed coat [26]. A greater content of water means more substrate for photosynthesis, therefore greater energy production. On the other hand, with greater content of melanin, lignin, or tannin, the hitherto unknown water dissociative properties of these molecules would allow for more energy production by means of greater water splitting activity, so the seed would still have enough energy for germination. Germination could be defined as a series of orderly biochemical reactions, and each of these reactions requires energy in the first place.

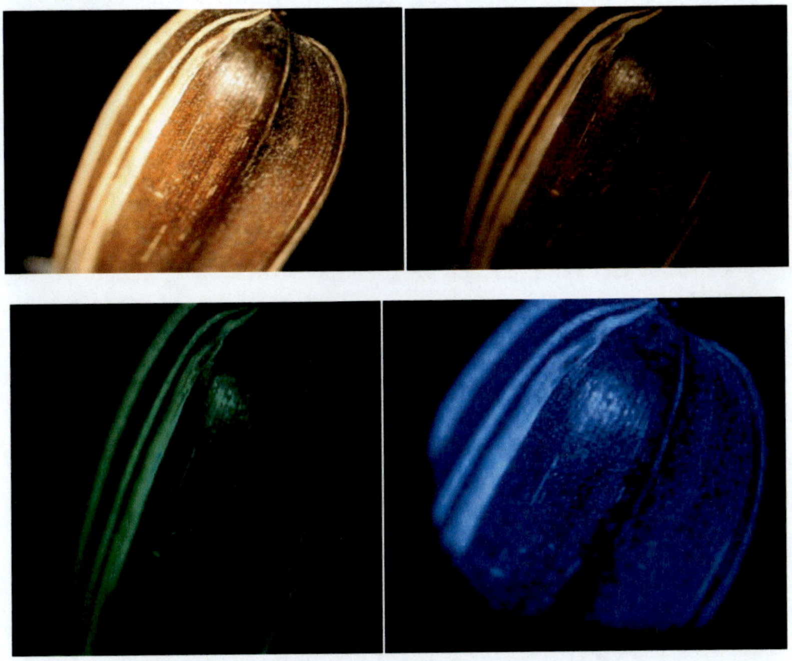

Figure 7. Sunflower seeds. Like melanin, lignin looks like a dark substance under all the different wavelengths used. Lignin, like melanin, absorbs a wide zone of the electromagnetic spectrum. The presence of melanin is doubtless.

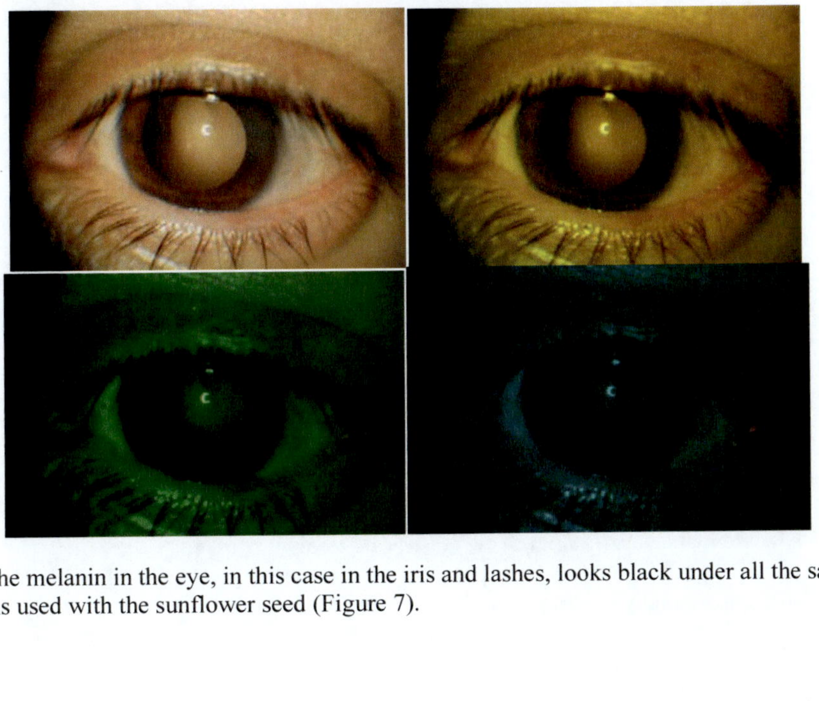

Figure 8. The melanin in the eye, in this case in the iris and lashes, looks black under all the same wavelengths used with the sunflower seed (Figure 7).

In other plant species, the color of the testa has been related to the content of tannin. Tannins are a very diverse family of poliphenolic compounds [27], as melanin and lignin are. They can subdivide into condensed and hydrolysable tannins, and both groups are capable of complexing with proteins, polysaccharides, and other macromolecules, as it occurs with melanin and lignin.

Tannins are not the only poliphenols that are found in seed coats. Lignin is also a poliphenolic constituent of the secondary walls of plant tissue. There is no lignin preparation (as it happens with melanin) that is devoid of other cell wall components.

Lignin and melanin are at all times closely present in tissues that normally have a high content of water. There are many similarities between both compounds; therefore we could say lignin is a type of melanin. The assumption that lignin has water dissociative properties, like melanin does, and its ever presence in the tree stem could explain the dynamics and physiology of the plant sap circulation, a well-known fact poorly understood until now.

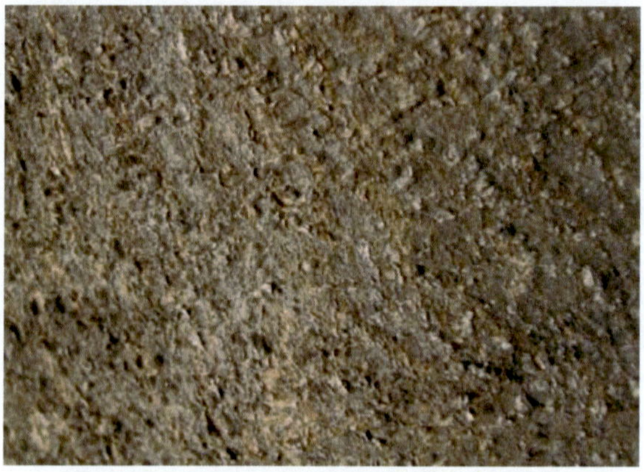

Figure 9. Photography of a tree cortex. Notice the resemblance of lignin with the image of Figure 10.

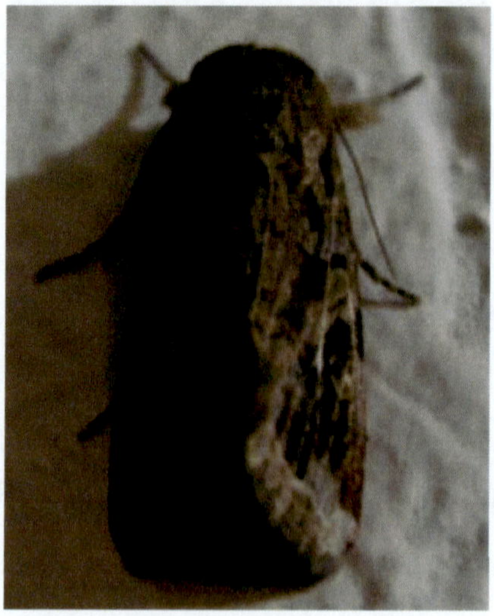

Figure 10. Microphotography of a moon moth; notice the resemblance of melanin with lignin in the tree cortex.

Table 1. Comparative table of the structure-properties-function relationship of Melanin, Lignin, and Tannin

	Melanin	Lignin	Tannin
Synthesized from	Phenylalanine	Phenylalanine	Phenylalanine
Presence in Nature	Widely	Widely	Widely
Formula	Unknown	Unknown	Unknown
Studies in Lab	Not possible or not conclusive	Not possible or not conclusive	Not possible or not conclusive
Main Function	Unknown	Unknown	Unknown
Kingdom	Animal and Plants	Plants	Plants
Studies *in vivo*	Extremely difficult	Extremely difficult	Extremely difficult
Water dissociation	Yes	Yes	Yes

From now on, glucose cannot be considered any more as source of energy. Glucose is mainly a source of biomass, and therefore it has an important role in structural and metabolic functions, as substrate only, not as source of energy. In this work, we explain several details about our unexpected and astonishing finding that will change, undoubtedly, several misconceptions about numerous metabolic processes.

Pigments in Nature

The great pigments of living things are the hemoglobins, chlorophylls, carotenoids, flavonoids and melanins [28]. The most neglected of these are the melanins, and not without reason. The prosthetic groups of the first four substances are orderly arrays of single and double bonds. Their proteins moieties are easily studied using conventional techniques. When melanins are isolated from living tissue, they produce an insoluble and amorphous mud that defies analysis by classical techniques.

The melanins are an important class of pigmentary macromolecules found throughout nature [29]. Eumelanin is the predominant form in humans and acts as the primary photoprotectant in our skin and eyes. Unique among biomacromolecules, the melanins are broadband UV and visible light absorbers. Their spectra display no chromophoric bands and follow a smooth single exponential dependence on wavelength, increasing monotonically towards the UV [30]. Most melanins are also chemically and photochemically very stable and are potent free radical scavengers and antioxidants. In a more general sense, the broader structure-property-function relationships that dictate the behavior of these important biological macromolecules are still poorly understood [31]. In particular, major questions still remain concerning the basic structural unit [32].

Paul Meredith et al., have been working in their laboratory over the past few years. Their work has concentrated on understanding these important properties with respect to natural melanins and tailored synthetic analogues. Their application-focused work is part of a broader program of condensed matter physics, synthetic organic chemistry, quantum chemistry, and molecular biophysics aimed at gaining a more complete understanding of melanin structure-property-function relationships. In spite of all their hard work, these researchers have not detected the hitherto unknown capability of melanin to dissociate and reform the water molecule because a test tube never will react to elevated concentrations of hydrogen and diatomic oxygen, a key difference with my work, where circumstantially we could detect the biological effects of both elements in retinal tissue *in vivo.*

Several steady-state photoluminescence studies have demonstrated that melanins possess an extremely low radiative quantum yield (i.e., the fraction of excitation photons that ultimately lead to a spontaneously emitted photon) [33]. Meredith et al. recently reported the first accurate measurement of yield for a synthetic eumelanin and found it to be $<6x10^{-4}$, i.e., 99.94% of absorbed photon energy is dissipated non-radiatively [34].

In conclusion, in the lab, there is no data that could suggest or at least lead researchers to think that melanin is in humans the analogue to chlorophyll in plants.

Melanin synthesis occurs in specialized organelles called melanosomes, and in tissues like skin they could migrate transcellularly. The migration of the keratinocytes and melanosomes results in a pigment gradient with a maximum melanin concentration toward the base of the epidermis. This inverted umbrella-like structure has led to much speculation regarding the efficacy of melanin as a sunscreen; however, in light of our findings on the role melanin plays in the production of energy, the topsy-turvy configuration is much more understandable.

The location of melanins in obscure internal body sites, their exotic chemical an physical properties, the sequestering of the pigment in protective subcellular particles, and the disease states resulting from absence of melanin all lead to speculation that melanins must have other functions than the simple solar protection. This sunscreen dogma is based primarily on the fact that people with dark skin are resistant to sunburn.

Between several proposed functions for Melanin, we have:

- Melanin acts as camouflage and adornment.
- Melanin is a sunscreen.
- Melanin is a radical scavenger.
- Melanin is a Photo and Radio-sensitizer.
- Melanin binds to drugs.
- Melanin transforms one kind of energy into another.

There has been a great deal published that melanin can transform light energy into electrical energy and heat [35], and detailed published observations on birds, for example, that pecten, a strange intra-ocular organ with unresolved function(s), is much enlarged and heavily melanized in birds fighting gravity, hypoxia, thirst and hunger during long-distance, frequently sub-zero, non-stop migration, may help cope with energy and nutrient needs under extreme conditions, by a marginal but critical, melanin-initiated conversion of light to metabolic energy, coupled to local metabolite recycling [36]. Our own unpublished observations, however, about feathers in birds is that the arrangement of their structure allows birds to absorb atmospheric humidity in a way that there is no resultant moisture, and the droplets of water are collected through superficial channels of the barb inside the central space of the rachis, creating a flow of water that through the hollow shaft, or calamus, can reach the skin of the bird where the melanin can make the process of water dissociation, allowing the bird to transform photonic energy into chemical energy. This allows the migrating bird to fly during long hours, or even during days, without losing weight in spite of the fact that migrating species fly without drinking and eating at all. We must remember that in the presence of low levels of glucose in the blood, the Krebs cycle can go into reverse.

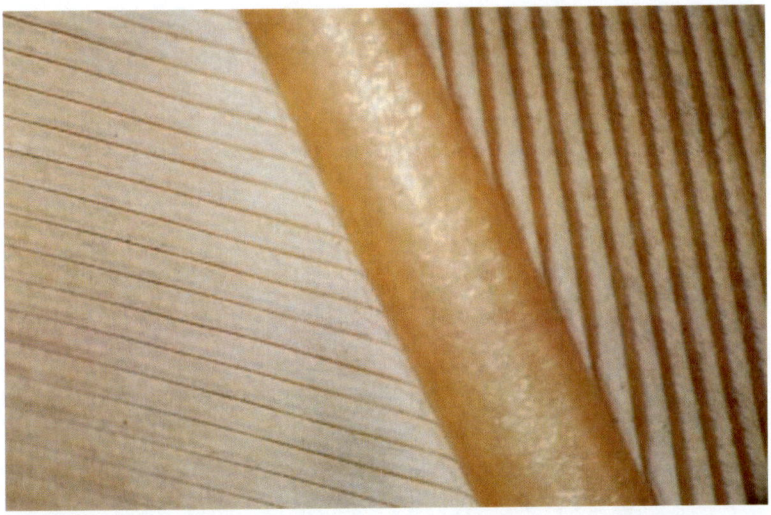

Figure 11. Bird's Feather. Magnification 40 X. (Solís-Herrera, 2011) Notice the channels formed in the barb, with a disposition that drives the water droplets formed by atmospheric moisture due to the movement of the feather during the bird's flight. Condensed moisture is directed to the hollow shaft or calamus, where water is collected and brought in contact with the skin of the bird, allowing melanin to transform photonic energy into chemical energy by means of melanin's water dissociation capability.

HUMAN PHOTOSYNTHESIS, THE STORY

Nobody before us described or wrote about the astonishing capacity of melanin to split the water molecule, like plants do through chlorophyll, and yet, our chlorophyll analogue, melanin is much more efficient [37].

Our findings came as a result of a twelve-year study with the aim to improve treatments for the three main causes of blindness. Initially, our main focus was in the observation of retinal blood vessels in living patients. However, the strategy to enhance as much as possible several and significant details of the blood vessels, their shape, size, direction, etc., gave us the unexpected finding that melanin detection was also improved, and thus its omnipresence made more evident.

Thereafter, the structure-property-function and relationship of melanin and its interaction with the retinal and choroid blood vessels gradually and powerfully drew our attention. In fact, the very important interplay between both tissues was detected early, at most three months after initiating our study, and after that, melanin became the main variable in our study. We started in 1990, however, twelve years were necessary to get a complete understanding of the main role that marvelous compound called melanin has in the recollection or harvesting of photonic energy present constantly in the environment in the form of electromagnetic waves of different sizes or wavelength and frequency, and the subsequent dissociation/re-association of the water molecule by the melanin via this harvested energy.

$$2H_2O \longrightarrow 2H_2 + O_2$$ Plants

$$2H_2O \longleftrightarrow 2H_2 + O_2$$ Humans

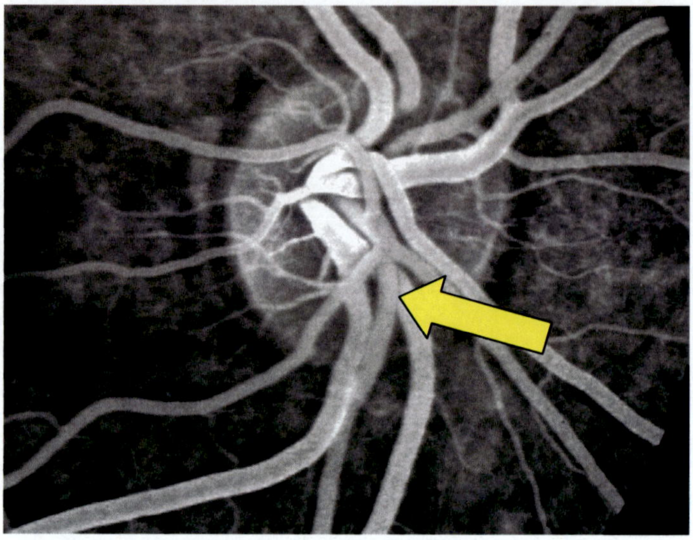

Figure 12. Optic Nerve of the right eye. The capillaries of the optic nerve are well delineated, taking into account that the normal diameter of the nerve is circa 1,200 microns. Melanin is indicated by the arrowhead (Solís-Herrera, 1998).

ATP is not a source of energy; instead, it is a complex system that absorbs energy from the photosynthesis process, acting more like a regulator. In accordance with our findings, when ATP is broken and ADP is formed, energy is absorbed, not released. The opposite happens when ADP is transformed to ATP, energy is then released.

Skin as an Example in the Human Body

The skin is the only organ besides the lungs that is directly exposed to atmospheric oxygen. The superficial layer, the epidermis, has no vasculature [38]. As early as 1851, Gerlach [39] was able to show that human skin takes up oxygen from the atmosphere. However, several reports in the field are coherent with the fact that the skin, as any cell, organ, and system, can split the water molecule and therefore produce oxygen *in situ.*

Until now, it has not been possible to determine the thickness of the layer (T) that characterizes the contribution of the so-called transcutaneous oxygen flux to the total skin oxygen supply. This is perhaps due to the fact that the main source of energy for the cell is the hydrogen, not the oxygen; oxygen is toxic at any concentration. Therefore, the search for levels of oxygen has proven to be very difficult, and the results have been, at best, random; thus, this search does not make much sense at all. On the other hand, changes in the oxygen absorption caused by increased or decreased blood flow cannot be detected, a fact that is astonishing according to the traditional theory that the main source of oxygen is blood flow. However, if we take into account the process of human photosynthesis, we can understand this is not the case, given that the main source of oxygen in blood is in fact produced by human photosynthesis.

The invasive measurements introduce several confusing factors, e.g., the needle puncture probably produces a local hyperemia increasing the oxygen supplied by the blood. However, demonstrated penetration depth of atmospheric oxygen in the upper 100 um seems that the diffusion of oxygen can only be from the skin surface and not from the blood to the skin surface.

However, in their studies, researchers rarely take into account the amount of melanin present in the skin. In all the experiments performed by Dr. Stücker [Ref. [38], an increase of transcutaneous oxygen flux was observed during induced ischemia, and the removal of capillary oxygen from the skin was negligible. We must turn to the role of water dissociation in the skin (human photosynthesis), because it explains very well these apparent contradictory results. In reality, the main source of oxygen is the generation in situ by means of the water dissociation process and not by the blood flow. Furthermore, it has been found that the determination of the decrease in Po_2 after stopping the oxygen supply is strongly temperature dependent. At 43 °C Vo_2 =4700 ml O_2 m^{-3} min^{-1} was derived from $tcPo_2$ measurements. At about 35 °C, an oxygen uptake value of 1470 ml 0_2 m^{-3} min^{-1} has been measured with intradermal needle electrodes. From the perspective of human photosynthesis, the infrared wavelengths are a kind of energy that could be absorbed by the photosystem and the transduction is increased.

Under normal conditions, the upper skin layers are supplied exclusively by the diffusion of oxygen from the atmosphere. This assumption is wrongly justified by the observation of only small changes of $tcJo_2$ during occlusion. In reality, the epidermis, as every other tissue, is strongly dependent on the products that result from the Human Photosynthesis process, which means Hydrogen and Oxygen, both diatomic.

Experiments using polarographic Po_2 needle electrodes have revealed characteristics of the intracutaneous Po_2 profiles; the Po_2 decreases continuously from a maximum at the skin surface—the area with exposure at most with electromagnetic radiations and therefore higher levels of photosynthesis in the region—to the upper layers of the papillary dermis until reaching a minimum, followed by a slight increase in the deeper skin layers, where the oxygen transported through the blood flow has a more significant role.

Dr. Stücker reached the conclusion that the measurements made during their experiments indicate that the capillary contribution to the oxygen supply of the corium is very limited. Other facts that show the importance of the human photosynthesis process is that the oxygen permeability of tissue is strongly dependent upon water content [40]. If the tissue has more water, then the water dissociation could increase due to the higher availability of the substrate itself.

Researchers say that the whole epidermis and the upper corium can therefore be supplied with oxygen from the atmosphere but more exactly by the human photosynthesis. It has been shown that under normal conditions, atmospheric oxygen can supply the upper skin layers to a depth of 0.25-0.40 mm. This is three to ten times deeper that had been calculated previously by Fitzgerald [41] in 1957, and Baumgärtl [42] in 1987. The difference is too large to think in methodological differences, but if we take into account the unexpected ability of the human tissue to split the water molecule and therefore produce oxygen and mainly hydrogen in situ, the differences are much more understandable. This may have significant consequences with regards to the treatment of lesions such as venous and ischemic ulcers.

Melanin splits the water molecule in diatomic oxygen and hydrogen, as chlorophyll does in plants; inspired by this analogy and with the main objective of attracting attention to the fact that in the very first step, both photosynthesis in plants and in humans (and therefore mammals) is identical, we decided to name this process "Human Photosynthesis."

In accordance with manmade classifications: plant kingdom and animal kingdom are then both photoautotrophic when we take into account the existence of the hitherto unknown water dissociation capability of melanin, that we named "human photosynthesis" because of the analogy.

The impact of this new knowledge in several fields of science is undoubtedly enormous.

REFERENCES

[1] Hall, David O., Rao, K.K., *Photosynthesis*, 6th ed. 1999, reprinted 2011. Published by Cambridge University Press. Cambridge, UK.

[2] M. Neefs, Y. Van de Peer, P. De Rijk, S. Chapelle, R. De Wachter, *Nucleic Acids Res.* 21, 3025 (1993).

[3] Gupta, R.S., T. Mukhtar, and B. Singh. 1999. Evolutionary relationships among photosynthetic prokaryotes (Heliobacterium chlorum, Chloroflexus aurantiacus, cyanobacteria, Chlorobium tepidum and proteobacteria): implications regarding the origin of photosynthesis. *Molecular Microbiology* 32(5):893-906.

[4] Blankenship, Robert E. In the book: *Molecular Mechanisms of Photosynthesis.* Published by Blackwell Science, United Kingdom 2002.

[5] Dau, Holger, Haumann, Michael. Eight Steps Preceding O-O Bond Formation in Oxygenic Photosynthesis -A Basic Reaction Cycle of the Photosystem II Manganese Complex. SCI-BIO, *Photosynthesis-Energy from the Sun.* 2008.

[6] Jin Xiong, William M. Fischer, Kazuhito Inoue, Masaaki Nakahara, and Cari E. Bauer *Molecular Evidence for the Early Evolution of Photosynthesis.* Science 8 September 2000: 1724-1730. [DOI:10.1126/science.289.5485.1724]

[7] Rafhavendra, Agepati S., Govindjee. In chapter 1: Sir Jagadish Chandra Bose, Vol 32; C4 Photosynthesis and Related C02 Concentrating Mechanisms; of the series: *Advances in Photosynthesis and Respiration.* Edited by: Govindjee and Thomas D. Sharkey. Published by Springer, The Netherlands. 2011. ISBN 978-90-481-9406-3.

[8] Boyd et al., Vol. 315 no. 5812 pp. 612-617. *Science* 2 February 2007.

[9] Bowes, G., Ogren, W.L., and Hageman, R.H. (1971). Phosphoglycolate production catalyzed by ribulose diphosphate carboxylase. *Biochem. Biophys. Res. Commun.* 45, 716–722; Ogren, WL, Bowes, G., 1971. Ribulose diphosphate carboxylase regulates soybean photorespiration. *Nat. New Biol.* 230, 159-160.

[10] Brown et al., 1974; Van et al., 1976; Bowes G, Salvucci ME (1989) Plasticity in the photosynthetic carbon metabolism of submersed aquatic macrophytes. *Aquat Bot* 34: 233-266.

[11] Madsen, T.V., Sand-Jensen, K., 1991. Photosynthetic carbon assimilation in aquatic macrophytes. *Aquat. Bot.* 41, 5–40.

[12] Eighmy, T.T., Jahnke, L.S., Fagerberg, W.R., 1991. Studies of Elodea nuttallii grown under photorespiratory conditions: II. Evidence for bicarbonate active transport. Plant Cell Environ. 14, 157–166., Maberly SC, Madsen TV. 2002. Freshwater angiosperm carbon concentrating mechanisms: processes and patterns. *Functional Plant Biology* 29: 393–405.

[13] Madsen, J.D., J.A. Bloomfield, J.W. Sutherland, L.W. Eichler, and C.W. Boylen. 1996. The aquatic macrophyte community of Onondaga Lake: Field survey and plant-growth bioassays of lake sediments. *Lake and Reservoir Management* 12: 73–79.

[14] Sage Rowan F. Atmospheric CO2, *environmental stress and the evolution of C4 photosynthesis*. Volume 161, Issue 2, pages 341–370, February 2004.

[15] Van TK, Haller WT, Bowes G (1976) Comparison of the photosynthetic characteristics of three submersed aquatic plants. *Plant Physiol* 58: 761-768; Bowes and Salvucci, 1989.

[16] L. Cegelski and J. Schaefer (2006), NMR determination of photorespiration in intact leaves using in vivo $^{13}CO_2$ labeling, *Journal of Magnetic Resonance* 178: 1-10.

[17] Hu, Thomas Q. *Chemical Modification, Properties, and Usage of Lignin*. Springer, 2002. ISBN 978-0- 306-46769-1.

[18] Whetten, Ross. Sederoff, Ron. Lignin Biosynthesis. The Plant Cell, Vol. 7, 1001-1013, July 1995 10 Gould, J. Michael. Characterization of Lignin in Situ by Photoacoustic Spectroscopy. *Plant Physiol.* (1982) 70, 1521-1525 0032-0889/82/70/1521/05.

[19] Sarkanen KV, Hergert HL (1971) Classification and distribution. In: Sarkanen KV, Ludwig CH (eds) *Lignins*. Wiley-Interscience, New York, pp 43–94.

[20] Atalla and Agarwal, 1985; Raman microprobe evidence for lignin orientation in the native state of woody tissue. *Science* 227:636-638.

[21] Agarwal and Atalla, 1986 In-situ Raman microprobe studies of plant cell walls: macromolecular organization and compositional variability in the secondary wall of Picea mariana (mill.) *B.S.P. Planta* 169: 325-332.

[22] Lewis, N.G., Newman, J. Just, G. and Ripmeister, J. (1987): Determination of bonding patterns of 13C specifically enriched dehydrogenatively polymerized lignin in solution and solid state. *Macromolecules* 20: 1752-1756.

[23] Therashima N 1990 A new mechanism for formation of a structurally ordered protolignin macromolecule in the cell wall of tree xylem. *J. Pul Pap. Sci.* 16:J150-J155.

[24] Pickett-Heaps, J. D. (1968): Xylem wall deposition. Radioautographic investigations using lignin precursors. *Protoplasma* 3: 55-64.

[25] Morrison, M., Ssiedu, E.A., Stuchbury, T., Powell, A.A. Determination of Lignin and Tannin Contents of Cowpea Seed Coats. *Annals of Botany* 76: 287-290< 1995.

[26] Morrison, M., Ssiedu, E.A., Stuchbury, T., Powell, A.A. Determination of Lignin and Tannin Contents of Cowpea Seed Coats. *Annals of Botany* 76: 287-290< 1995.

[27] Mueller-Harvey I., McAllan A.B., 1992. Tannins. Their biochemistry and nutritional properties. In: *Advances in plant cell biochemistry and biotechnology,* Vol. 1 (Morrison I.M., ed.). JAI Press Ltd., London (UK), pp. 151-217.

[28] Lili, Helene Z. The Function of Melanin or Six Blind People Examine an Elephant. *BioEssays*. Vol. 14, No. 1-January 1992, pp. 42- 56.

[29] G. Prota (1992) *Melanins and Melanogenesis.* Academic Press, San Diego, CA.

[30] M.L. Wolbarsht, A.W. Walsh and G. George, *Appl. Opt.* 20, 2184-2186 (1981).

[31] K. B. Stark, J.M. Gallas, G.W. Zajac, M. Eisnerand J.T. Golab, *J. Phys. Chem.* B107, 3061-3067 (2003).

[32] Z.W. Zajac, J.M. Gallas, J. Cheng, M. Eisner, S. C. Moss and A. E. Alvarado-Swaisgood, *Biochim. Biophys. Acta,* 1199, 271 -278 (1994).

[33] J. B. Nofsingerand J.D. Simón (2001), *Photochem. Photobiol.,* 74, 31-37 (2001).

[34] P. Meredith and J. Riesz, *Photochem. Photobiol.*, 79(2), 211-216 (2004).

[35] Crippa, P.R., Mazzini, A., Salmelli, D. (1979). Oxidation of NADH by melanin: Effect of UV light and cooperions. *Physiol. Chem. Phys.* 11,491-499.

[36] Goodman, Geoffrey, Bercovich, Dani. Melanin directly converts light for vertebrate metabolic use: Heuristic thoughts on birds, Icarus and dark human skin. *Med Hypotheses.* 2008 May 12; 18479839 (P,S,E,B,D).

[37] Solís-Herrera, Arturo, Arias Esparza, Marta del Carmen, Solís -Arias Ruth I., Solís -Arias Paola E., Solís -Arias, Martha P. The unexpected capacity of melanin to dissociate the water molecule fills the gap between the Life before and after ATP. *Biomedical Research* 2010; 21 (2):224-226.

[38] Stücker, M. Struk, A. Altmeyer, P., Herde, M. The cutaneous uptake of atmospheric oxygen contributes significantly to the oxygen supply of human dermis and epidermis. *Journal of Physiology* (2002), 538, 3, pp. 985-994. DOI: 101013/physiology 2001.013067.

[39] Gerlach A. Über das Hautathmen. *Archives of Anatomy and Physiology.* 1851:431–479.

[40] Vaupel P. Effect of percental water content in tissue and liquids on the diffusion coefficients of O2, CO2, N2, H2. *Pflügers Archiv.* 1976; 361:201–204.

[41] Fitzgerald LR. Cutaneous respiration in man. *Physiological Reviews.* 1957; 37:325–345.

[42] Baumgärtl H, Ehrly AM, Saeger-Lorenz K, Lübbers DW. Initial results of intracutaneous measurements of PO2 profiles. In: Ehrly AM, Hauss J, Huch R, editors. *Clinical Oxygen Pressure Measurement.* Berlin: Springer; 1987. pp. 121–128.

In: Vegetable Consumption and Health: New Research
Editors: Claudia Wilson and Melinda Morree
ISBN: 978-1-62100-941-2

Chapter 4

DEVELOPMENT AND IMPLEMENTATION OF ENVIRONMENTALLY BENIGN APPROACHES FOR INTEGRATED PEST MANAGEMENT OF CRUCIFEROUS CROPS IN CHINA

Minsheng You[1,*], Youming Hou[1], Guang Yang[1], and Geoff Gurr[2]

[1]Institute of Applied Ecology, Fujian Agriculture and Forestry University, Fuhzou, China
[2]Faculty of Sciences, Charles Sturt University, Orange New South Wales, Australia

ABSTRACT

Cruciferous vegetables are one of the dominant food crops, and widely considered to be healthy foods containing multiple nutrients and phytochemicals. In China, cruciferous crops are mainly infested by lepidopteran, coleopteran and hemipteran pests, causing damage through the loss of crop yield or quality. Pest control has relied heavily on the application of chemical pesticides for a long time but many problems are associated with their use such as the appearance of resistant strains of pests and harmful effects on non-target organisms. To achieve better control of pests in cruciferous crops, efforts since the 1990s have been focused on developing and implementing integrated pest management (IPM) incorporating various environmentally benign approaches, including cultural practices, conservation biological control and behavioral regulation. The IPM system was designed as a flexible framework to minimize adverse effects on vegetable products, non-target species and environment, to maximize profit for growers, and to be sustainable. Over the past two decades, this IPM program has been extensively used to effectively control the major insect pests in cruciferous crops in the southern provinces of China, and proved to be ecologically sound, economically feasible, environmentally acceptable, and practically applicable.

* Corresponding author: Minsheng You, Institute of Applied Ecology and Research Center for Biodiversity and Eco-Safety, Fujian Agriculture and Forestry University, Fuzhou 350002, China. Tel: +86 591 83789396; Fax: +86 591 83768251, Email: msyou@iae.fjau.edu.cn.

Keywords: Cruciferous vegetable, habitat management, biological control, mating disruption, repellent agent, blinding trap

INTRODUCTION

Cruciferous vegetables, especially cabbage, kale, mustard and radish, are important foods in people's daily lives. In China, cruciferous vegetables are planted on approximately 8.7 million hectares of land every year and account for about half of the total area and yield of vegetables. Thus, these vegetables play pivotal roles in boosting farmer income, augmenting agricultural efficiency and promoting the export of agricultural products. However, the production of cruciferous vegetables is plagued by many pests that often inflict heavy losses on yield and quality. The extent of output reduction can reach 30%-60%; occasionally, no produce can be harvested. In southern China, where climate and cultural conditions are suitable for many insects, the occurrence of and damage from infestations are even more severe, with the greatest loss caused by the diamondback moth (*Plutella xylostella*), the striped flea beetle (*Phyllotreta striolata*), noctuid moths (primarily the Oriental leafworm moth, *Spodoptera litura*) and the beet armyworm (*S. exigua*). These insects pose a great challenge for pest control.

Since the late 1980s, the simple nature of the cruciferous vegetable agroecosystem combined with heavy reliance on chemical pesticides led to biodiversity reduction in vegetable fields and the problems of "3Rs" (i.e., residues, resurgence and resistance), manifesting a vicious cycle of rampant infestation, pesticide inundation, chemical deposition (in vegetables) and re-infestation. Therefore, this cycle has become a key issue in safe vegetable production, which requires solving. In China and elsewhere, previous studies on the occurrence patterns and control technologies for vegetable pests have traditionally focused on individual technologies while overlooking the biological community of the field and adjacent areas. This is exemplified in reports on controlling *P. xylostella* using vegetable varieties and planting arrangement (Talekar and Sheton, 1993); granulosis virus (Lü, 1998); parasitoid wasps (He, 1998); and the application of *Bt* toxin from *Bacillus thuringiensis* (Wang et al., 2006). Likewise, studies on the control of *P. striolata* mostly examined one particular technology such as resistant plant varieties (Amano, 1984), the introduction and utilization of parasitoid wasps (Wykie, 1984);and the use of entomopathogenic nematodes (Zhang, 1998). Equivalent examples of *S. litura* control include the use of *Telenomus remus* Nixon (Joshi et al., 1982); *Bt* (Jiang and Deng, 1997); and entomopathogenic nematodes (Wang and Li, 1994). Importantly, several reports discuss the application of nuclear polyhedrosis virus, which has entered the commercial production stage. These species-oriented studies play an extremely important role in effectively containing the damage from principal field pests and depressing their population densities.Work since the early 1990s has focused on controlling the most damaging pests (*P. xylostella L., P. striolata* and *Spodoptera* spp.) with fewer pesticides and increased vegetable safety, focusing on the specific areas described below. First, we examine the damage processes and mechanisms of the major pests and elucidate the underlying causes of infestations. Second, control technologies, including habitat management, biological control, behavioral modulation, disorienting prevention and pesticide reduction measures are reviewed. Finally, key technologies are integrated to develop a management system targeting the major pests which is then evaluated in the field. Thus, this chapter details a non-chemical management system for the major cruciferous vegetable pests which is the culmination of a 20-year effort.

1. Patterns in Population Development and Eruptive Growth of the Major Cruciferous Vegetable Pests

From the perspective of the regional agro-landscape and the cruciferous ecosystem, we studied and elucidated the interactions between individual functional groups in arthropod communities from different origins (within a vegetable field and between a vegetable field and a non-vegetable field). As expected, diversified vegetable fields harbored communities whose richness and Shannon-Wienner's (1949) diversity increased by 360.9% and 128.5%, respectively (You and Xu, 2000; Hou *et al.*, 2000a); arthropod species and natural enemies were increased by 12.8% and 39.5% (Figure 1), respectively. More importantly, the control efficacy of predatory functional groups was elevated by 65.5% (Xu and You, 1999; Cai *et al.*, 2007). In addition, a pesticide moratorium was followed by an increase of the general control index of natural enemies from 1.94 to 11.17 and a 3.3-fold increase in predator control efficacy (Hou *et al.*, 2000a; Hou *et al.*, 2000c).By overcoming the limitations of mass rearing *P. striolata* in the laboratory (Liu et al., 2009), we were able to uncover the mechanisms of its population fluctuation and eruptive growth from a variety of perspectives, such as pesticide resistance (Fu *et al.*, 2004; Fu *et al.*, 2006; Zheng *et al.*, 2009), differentiation of geographic populations (Fu *et al.*, 2008) and host plants (Liu and You, 2008). We demonstrated that desensitization of acetylcholinesterase was a major cause leading to the resistance to organophosphate and carbamate insecticides (Figure 2).In addition, termination of insecticide application reduced the population trend index from 5.28 to 1.86. The genomic variability among different geographic populations may influence their damage and eruptive growth. Furthermore, the host plants had tremendous effects on the larval development period, adult longevity and fecundity.

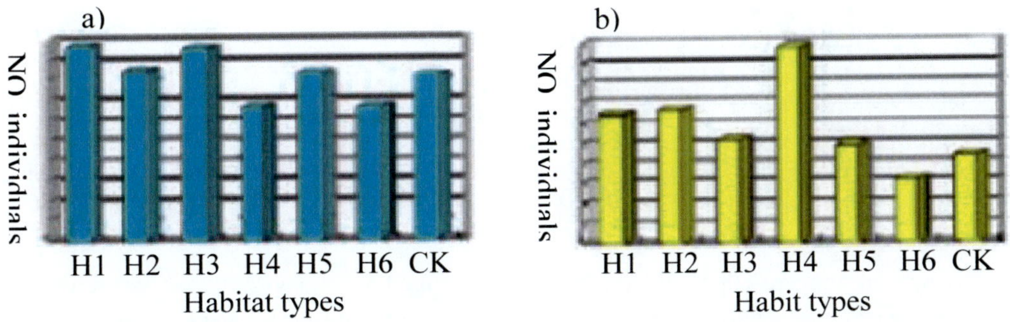

Figure 1. Individual numbers of herbivores and parasitoids in different vegetable habitats (H1-H6 denote habitats with different diversity, CK denotes the simplified habitat; a) herbivores; b) parasitoids).

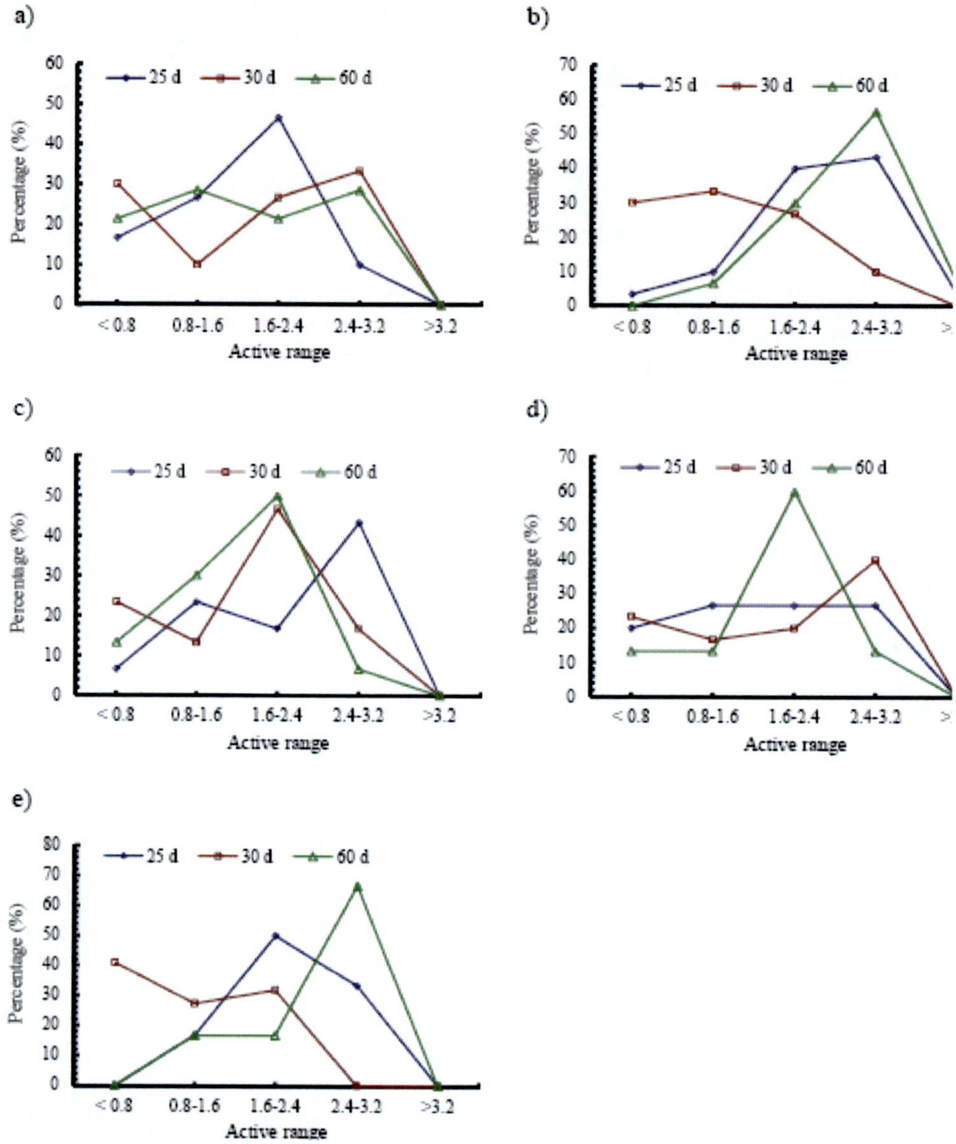

Figure 2. Distribution frequency of total esterase activity of *Phyllotreta striolata* adults feeding on different host plants (Fu, 2010); a) *Brassica campestris* L.ssp.*chinensis* (L.); b) *Brassica parachinensis* Bailey; c) *Brassica oleracea* L.var.*capitata* (L.); d) *Raphanus stativas*(L.); e) *Brassica campestris* L.ssp.

However, the growth of host plants also resulted in changes in pest preference; the general descending order of *P. striolata* preference was mustard, carrot, cabbage, Chinese cabbage and kale. Regarding *P. xylostella*, we evaluated the mechanisms of its population development and eruptive growth by dissecting several factors, including planting system (You *et al*., 2003), chemical pesticides (Liu and You, 1998, 2003; Hou *et al*., 2003), pest fitness and the triangle dynamics of vegetable-pest-natural enemy (You and Yang, 2001; Lü *et al*., 2004 ; Yang *et al*., 2004a).

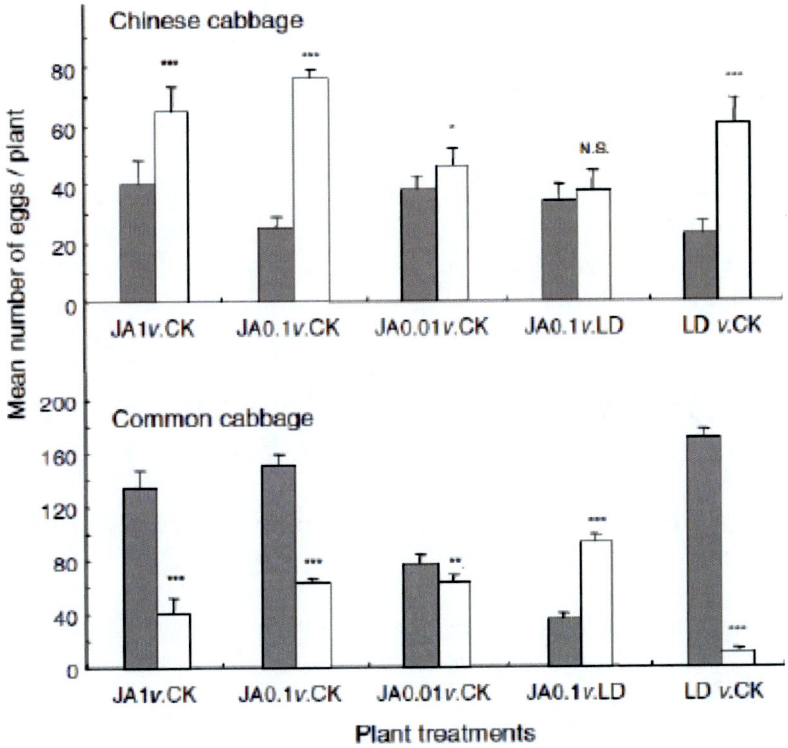

Figure 3. Number of eggs laid by female *Plutella xylostella* moths when they were provided with a choice of a relevant untreated control plant and a treated Chinese cabbage plant or a treated common cabbage. JA1, JA0.1 and JA0.01 indicate plants that received an application of 1 μmol mL-1, 0.1μmol mL-1or 0.01μmol mL-1jasmonic acid solution, respectively, LD indicates plants with larval damage and CK indicates intact plants. See text for test details, and see Table 3 for results of statistical analysis. (Lüet al., 2004.

We found that large-scale cultivation of cruciferous vegetables was associated with a 2.6- to 3.8-fold annual increase of the *P. xylostella* population trend index. However, a pesticide moratorium was followed by the reduction of the *P. xylostella* population trend index from 36.27 to 5.32.

By cloning and expressing the myrosinase gene from the flowering Chinese cabbage (Zao 49) in a variety of hosts, we found that myrosinase expression reduced the fitness of vegetables to *P. xylostella* (Yang *et al*., 2011). In addition, host plants underwent a change of volatile release after being foraged on and damaged by *P. xylostella*, resulting in their significantly enhanced attractiveness to the parasitoid *Cotesia plutellae* and increased search capacity of the wasp (Yang et al., 2004b).

P. xylostella adults exhibited increased preference for kale but decreased attraction to cabbage when the two vegetables were treated with exogenous jasmonic acid (Figure 3). These results indicate that the host plants harbor a mechanism to balance constitutive defense and induced defense (Lü and Liu, 2004, 2005).We also investigated the population dynamics and eruptive growth of *S. exigua*considering the host plant (Si *et al*., 2005) and pesticide resistance (Si *et al*., 2001; He *et al*., 2003). We discovered that the pests occurred annually in southern China (6-10 generations each year), had considerable overlapping generations and displayed no apparent overwintering phenomenon. *Spodopters exigua* exhibited a wide host range. In summer, even when there was minimal cruciferous vegetable acreage, the *S. exigua* population remained at a considerable size that could cause severe damage. Furthermore, the *S. exigua* population displayed a high level of resistance to many pesticides, including organo phosphorus and synthetic pyrethroids.

The maximal resistance was reported to be 2912- to 4564-fold (Zou and Si, 1996). It has also been shown that an important mechanism of *S. exigua*poisoning is the inhibition of carboxylesterase and acetylcholinesterase activities in larvae (Table 1) (Zhu *et al.*, 1996; Zhu *et al.*, 2007; Zhou *et al.*, 2009).

2. Habitat Management and Biological Control for the Major Cruciferous Vegetable Pests

2.1. Habitat Management to Conserve Natural Enemies of Major Vegetable Pests

We examined the correlation between biodiversity in the regional agricultural landscape and spatial/temporal dynamics of field arthropod communities. Additionally, we evaluated the control processes and efficacy of the biodiversity-harboring ecosystems of vegetable fields and habitat management on the major pests.

Table 1. Effects of insecticide treatment on carboxylesterase activity of *Spodoptera exigua*larvae (He *et al.*, 2003)

Insecticide	Dose /mg·L^{-1}	Mortality /%	Enzyme activity /OD_{600}(mg Pr·min)$^{-1}$	Suppression Rate /%
Cypermethrin	1000	13.33	1.54 ± 0.19	61.83
Methomyl	1200	45.45	1.14 ± 0.13	71.90
Acephate	3000	9.09	0.28 ± 0.02	93.12
Chlor Fluazuron	50	53.33	1.60 ± 0.00	60.56
Chlorpyrifos	1000	52.38	0.21 ± 0.01	94.69
Control (Check)			4.05 ± 0.24	—

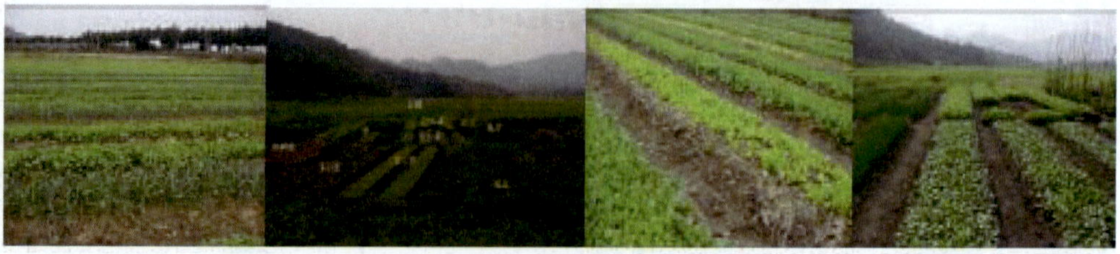

Figure 4. Intercropping manipulation for habitat management of major insects in cruciferous fields.

On this basis, we established habitat management techniques in which natural enemies are conserved and utilized to control major pests, including a variety of measures such as landscape layout, intercropping, paddy-upland rotation and fallow land (You *et al.*, 2004). Intercropping was facilitated by sandwiching one plot of garlic or spring vegetables with two plots of cruciferous vegetables or by flanking one plot of cruciferous vegetables with two plots (20 cm wide) of garlic or spring vegetables (Figure 4).

Such measures resulted in species diversity indices of 4.09 and 4.07, respectively, and a dominant concentration index of 0.09 in the vegetable fields. During the growth period from the seedling stage to the maturity stage, the numbers of individual natural enemies were sustained at high levels.This was most pronounced for the parasitoid Aphelinidae and Aphidiidae wasps and their natural predators, whose individual numbers increased by 36-87% (Cai *et al.*, 2010, 2011).For the first time, we found that wolf spiders predated *P. striolata* and that intercropping between garlic and Chinese cabbage augmented the populations of wolf spiders and cobweb spiders, resulting in an increase in predator species richness of 261% (Cai and You, 2007).

The major parasitoid natural enemies of *P. xylostella* include Cotesia *plutellae*, *Oomyzus sokolowskii*, *Trichogramma chilonis* and *Diadromus collaris*. The first two species are dominant in terms of parasitism rate and number, and *T. chilonis* was reported in the Fuzhou area for the first time.

Predatory natural enemies, such as *Erigonidium graminicolum*, *Theridion octomaculatum* and *Paederus fuscipes,* are most abundant in fields. However, *Clubiona japonicola*, carabid beetles, *Lycosa pseudoamulata* and *Misumenopos tricuspidata* are among the most effective predators (Wu and You, 2001). The intercropping between cruciferous vegetables and garlic reduced the population growth trend indices of *P. xylostella* and *P. striolata* by 5.3- and 3.7-fold, respectively.

2.2. Strip Application of Insect Pathogenic Nematodes

To fully tap the active search potential of *Steinernema* spp. nematodes in moist soil, we proposed a strip application technology, using *Steinernema* spp. to control the *P. striolata* population (Figure 5). The field density was decreased from 7.00 billion nematodes/ha in the inundated application to 1.75 billion/ha in the strip application. While the latter method still resulted in an infection rate of 71.3% on day 6 post-application (Table 2) (Hou *et al.*, 2001a, 2001b), such a technological improvement reduced cost by 75.0% while generating the same control efficacy.

2.3. Mass Rearing and Application of *Diadegma Semiclausum* Hellen

A dominant parasitoid wasp of *P. xylostella*, *D. semiclausum*, was successfully introduced from Taiwan (Figure 6) in 1997. Based on comprehensive studies of its biology and ecology, we developed a series of technologies for mass propagation, field release and colonization of *D. semiclausum* (Chen *et al.*, 2000; Chen *et al.*, 2001a). A self perpetuating population has been successfully established in highland vegetable-growing areas in Yunnan Province, which now has a parasitism rate of 20.0-40.0% and a maximum rate of 74.7%. This is superior to the impact of two local dominant parasitoid wasps, *Orientohmiteles sp.* (24.0%) and *C. plutellae* (21.5%) (Chen *et al.*, 2001b; Chen *et al.*, 2003).

The production cost of *D. semiclausum* is 120-150 Renminbi(approximately US$18)/ha. A single release could continuously and effectively contain the population growth of *P. xylostella* and could reduce pesticide use by 35.0%. As such, it saved chemical and labor costs equaling six-times the cost of the mass released *D. semiclausum.*

Table 2. Application techniques and their simulated effects on*Steinernema carpocapsae*

Striped flee beetle larvae number	Nematode dosage (ten thousand individual·m^{-2})	Number of strips	Infection rate(%)	Control effect(%)	Nematode dosage (hundred million individual·ha^{-1})
<0.5	70	3	72.59	82.3	17.5
0.5-1.0	70	3	72.85	82.7	17.5
1.0-1.5	70	3	73.39	71.8	17.5
1.5-2.0	60	4	70.29	87.8	20.0
>2.0	60	4	70.56	86.0	20.0

Note: The striped flee beetle larvae number is the individual number in the soil sampled by a soil sampler (h = 15 cm, d = 8 cm).

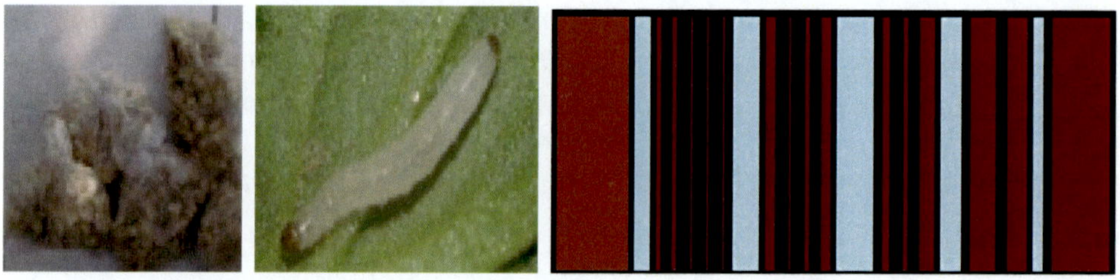

Figure 5. Sketch map of *Steinernema carpocapsae* and its strip-spraying in fields.

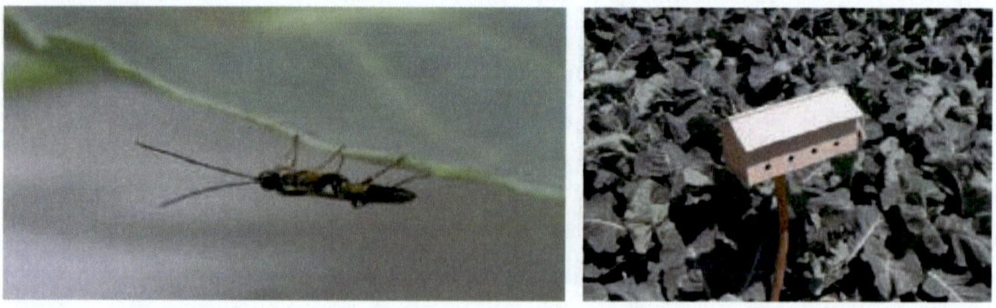

Figure 6. *Diadegma semiclausum*(left) and its container (right) for release in the fields.

2.4.Using *S. Exigua* Attractants to Induce Adults to Carry and Transmit Virus

Currently, many reports in China and abroad demonstrate that the transmission of insect viruses can be mediated by female insects (via their ovaries) (references). However, no study has been performed to examine if spermatozoa in males can mediate such a function. This project assessed the transmission (vertical and horizontal) routes and efficiency of viruses in populations of target pests (Jiang *et al.*, 2004; Zhou *et al.*, 2009).

Based on these results, we were able to take advantage of a feature of *Microplitis* spp.: the wasps prefer to parasitize aggregatory hosts of low instar larvae. This enabled us to create a novel method of employing the larval parasitoid wasps to transmit viruses. This method achieved control outcomes of 72.3%-88.2% (*S. litura*) and 81.5%-89.7% (*S. exigua*) (Figures 7 and 8) (Jiang *et al.*, 2005; Jiang *et al*, 2011). In addition, we discovered that the viruses may undergo vertical transmission via spermatozoa in males, which enabled us to pioneer a new technology (i.e., using attractants for both sexes to seduce adults harboring viruses), resulting in control efficacies of 90.2% (*S. litura*) and 89.7% (*S. exigua*), and a significant reduction of virus use by 85.0%.

Table 3. Evaluation of control effects of ethanol extracts from several heterologous plants on the diamondback moth

Ethanol extract from leaf and Stem(dry weight g/100ml)	Oviposition inhibition N_{0tr}/N_{0ck}	Egg hatching S_{Etr}/S_{0Ek}	Low-instar larvaeS_{STr}/S_{SCK}	IIPC
Eucalytus rubusta	0.30	0.58	0.31	0.05
Wedelia chinensis	0.49	0.63	0.36	0.11
Bidens pilosa	0.51	0.74	0.49	0.18
Lycopersicum esculentum	0.51	0.74	0.49	0.18
Polygonum hydropiper	0.50	0.82	0.46	0.19
Lantana camara	0.40	0.85	0.36	0.13
Citrus reticulata	0.44	0.86	0.67	0.27
Dicranopteris dichotoma	0.41	1.00	0.94	0.80

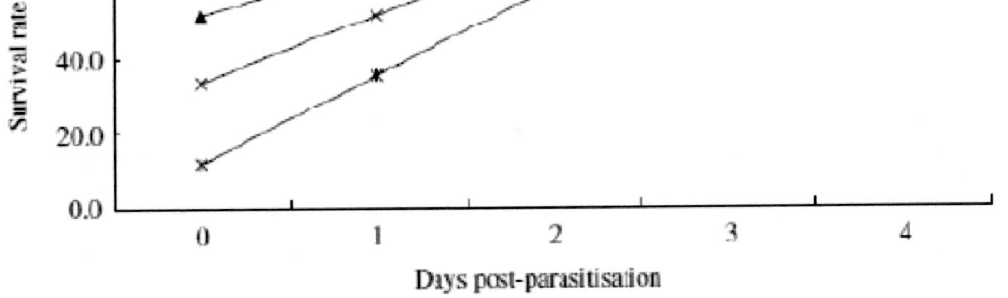

Figure 7. Survival rate of the parasitoid,*Microplitis pallidipes,* as affected by the time interval between exposure to the parasitoid and subsequent exposure to the virus and by virus concentration (logarithm). (Jiang et al, 2011).

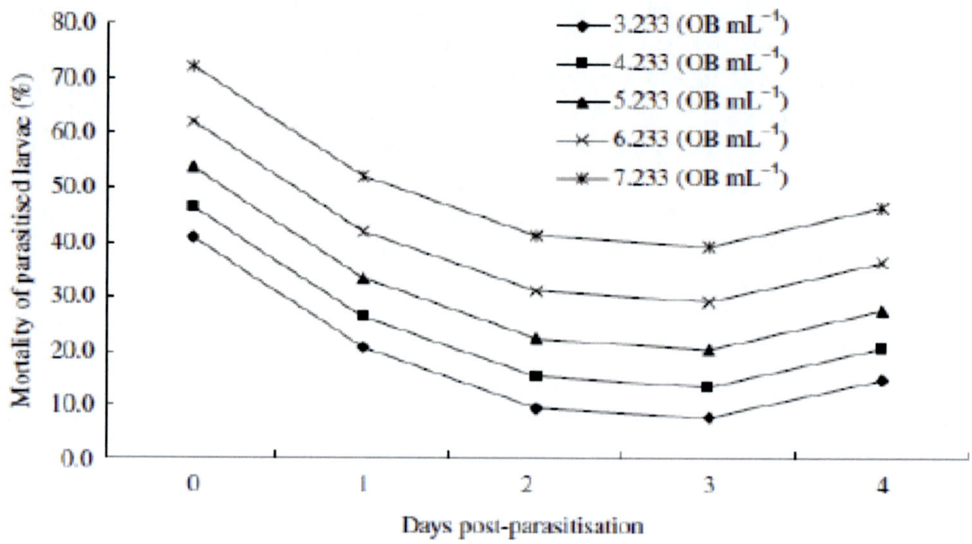

Figure 8. Mortality of parasitised larvae as affected by the time interval between exposure to the parasitoid and subsequent exposure to the virus and by virus concentration (logarithm).(iang et al, 2011).

3. Behavioral Modulation and Disorientation of Major Cruciferous Vegetable Pests

3.1. Yellow Sticky Trap for Control of *P. Striolata* Adults

It has been reported that *P. striolata* adults display the strongest preference for yellow and white colors, followed by green and blue (Fu *et al.*, 2004). Therefore, we developed a yellow sticky trap with a light wavelength of 585 nm reflected by the board (Figure 9). The optimum size of the floor board is 20 × 15 cm, and the squares above are 1 × 1 cm in size. The ingredients of the glue include colorless lubricant, butter or castor oil, rosin and paraffin. We succeeded in troubleshooting several glue problems, including anti-aging, anti-UV light and anti-flow issues.

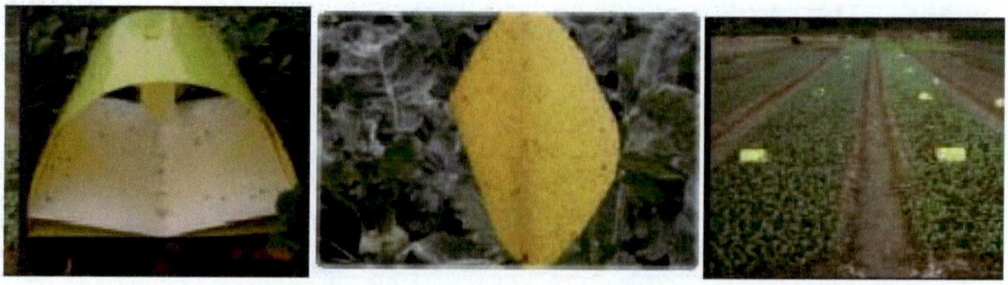

Figure 9. Yellowsticky traps for insects and their application in the fields.

Compared to similar products, our sticky trap has a trapping rate that is 3.6-fold greater, and the production cost is 30% lower. The sticky trap also made sampling, forecasting and surveying convenient (Fu *et al.*, 2005). The traps were applied at a density of 300/ha at a height of 2-3 cm over the plant canopy and were replaced every 30 d (3-fold longer than conventional products). The sticky trap exhibited excellent trapping outcomes for *P. xylostella*, leaf miners and whitefly (Lu *et al.*, 2003).

3.2. A New Type of LED Trapper for Control of *P. Xylostella*

Studies have shown that the light preference of *P. xylostella* follows a descending order of green, white, red, yellow and blue. Adults exhibit a particularly strong attraction toward green and white light on the first emergence day (Wan *et al.*, 2008). Hence, we developed a new type of*P. xylostella* Light Emitting Diode (LED) trapper that had a trapping rate enhanced by 38.2% compared to similar products (black light lamps and vibrational broad-spectrum insecticide lamps). As such, it reduced pesticide use by 42.0%. Additionally, it protected the natural enemies of Spodoptera spp. in the vegetable field (Zhao et al., 2008; Wan, 2008).

3.3. Applications of New Types of Sex Pheromone Agents and Traps

Our working team possesses the most comprehensive insect pheromone sources (> 300 compounds) in China and a unique strength in research of pheromone carriers, PVC microtubules and sticky pins. We improved pheromone ingredients and carrier types and developed microtubule trappers, boat-style trappers and hole-style trappers (Figure 10).

Together, these products sustain trapping of *P. xylostella* for 4 months (Figure 11) and improve the trapping rate by 75.0% with a reduction of costs by 1/3 (Hou *et al.*, 2000c, 2001d; Deng *et al.*, 2007). Currently, these products have been exported to South Korea, the United Arab Emirates, Saudi Arabia, the Philippines, Malaysia and Turkey.

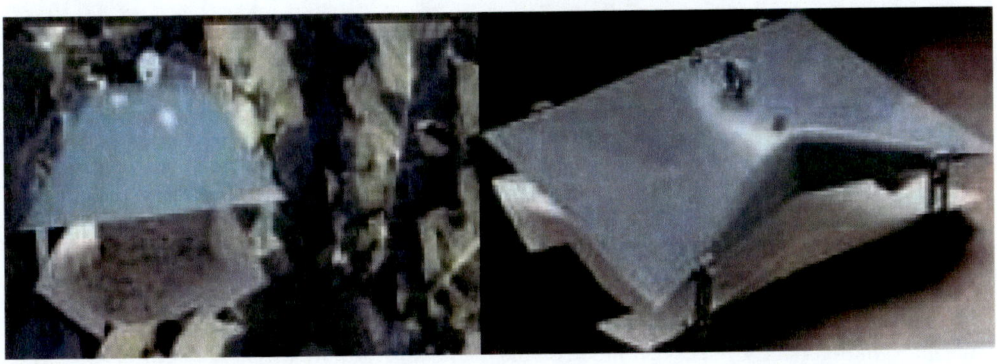

Figure 10. Moth trap and its application in the fields.

3.4. Development of Three Vegetable-Protecting Agents

Research into protective agents for vegetables in China and elsewhere is focused on plant compounds. Our studies took full advantage of the phenomenon that the secondary metabolites of heterologous plants strongly repel the major vegetable pests that migrate from exogenous habitats (or neighboring fields). In addition, we also examined the anti-feedant activities and contact toxicities of plant volatiles. This research collectively culminated in the establishment of a comprehensive control system, including assessment models and indices, for evaluating control outcomes (Hou, 2001). Specifically, we selected extracts from 36 plants (including tobacco, lotus, magnolia, bauhinia and forest red gum [*Eucalyptus tereticornis*]) that demonstrated prominent pest-control activities from the ethanol extracts of > 100 non-preferable plant species (Hou, 2001; Wei *et al.*, 2004, 2005; Yan *et al.*, 2005; Lai and You, 2005). We found that the main active ingredients of the essential oil from dragon juniper include (+)-epi-bicyclosesquiphellandrene and -cadinene, representing 13.7 and 6.3% of the total volume, respectively (Zhao and Hou, 2006).

The major active compounds in the 70% ethanol extract of Spanish flag (*Lantana camara*) are flavonoids, which account for 9.6 and 3.4% of the crude extracts (Hou *et al.*, 2001;Wei et al., 2004;2005;Yan et al., 2005; Lai and You, 2005). The ethanol extract of plume poppy (*Macleaya cordata*) demonstrates potent biological activities against *Pieris rapae*, *Colaphellus bowringi*, *Phaedon brassicae*, *P. striolata*, *Myzus persicae*,*S. litura* and *P. xylostella*; we identified two monomers from the plume poppy extract as protopine and allocryptopine (Zhang and You, 2008, 2009).

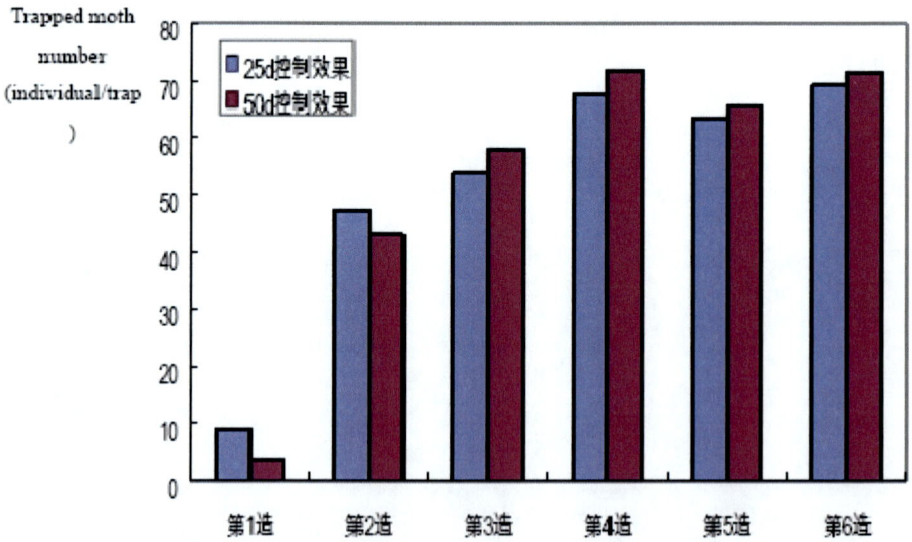

Figure 11. Control effects of sex pheromone on the diamondback moth in 6 continuous batches of vegetable fields.

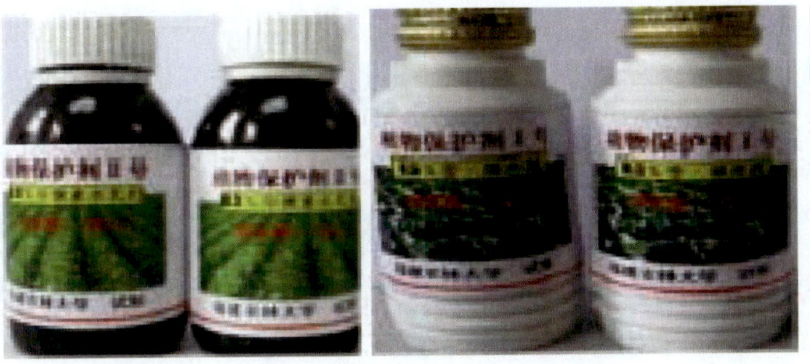

Figure 12.Protective agents for vegetables.

Moreover, we found that treatments of azadirachtin (5.0×10^{-3} ml/L), BIOACT-T35 (10.0 ml/L) and celangulin (10.0 ml/L) reduced the population trend index of *P. xylostella* to 2.27, 1.95 and 0.67, respectively. Finally, we developed three vegetable protective agents (Figure 12) that reduced pesticide use by ~50% (Hou *et al.*, 2002, 2003).

4. Using Tobacco Waste to Treat Soil for the Control of *P. Striolata*

Many reports indicate that tobacco waste can control pest behavior in many agro-systems, but similar studies have not been reported for the major vegetable pest *P. striolata*. This study involved sealing piles of tobacco waste (e.g., leaves and stems) for 2-3 months. Subsequently, the waste was chopped into small pieces, which were applied on the soil surface (2050 kg/ha). Seeds were then sown 12 h after plowing. Such a practice resulted in a 79.8% control rate for *P. striolata*, significantly higher than that of phoxim treatment (57.1%).

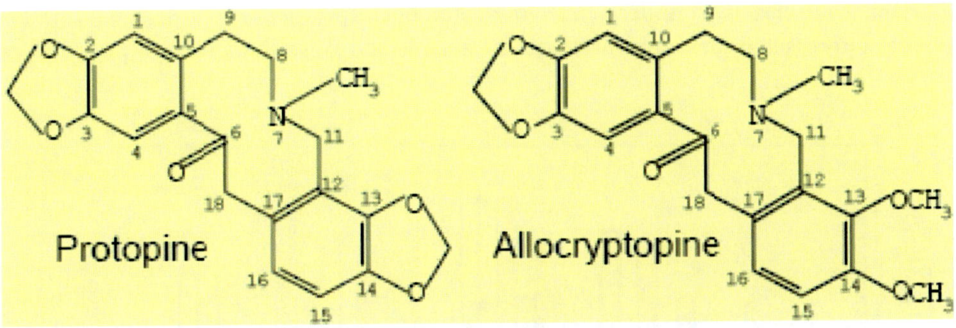

Figure 13. Chemical structure formula of the monomers in ethanol extract from *Macleya cordata.*

In addition, it reduced the population trend index of the pest below 1.882 (3.219 for phoxim treatment) and achieved a production retention rate of 77.1% (61.5% for phoxim treatment) (Figure 13, Table 4) (Hou *et al.*, 2000b). In the demonstration fields of three vegetables, such treatment excluded any use of pesticide and yielded a control rate of 79.8%

for *P. striolata* and a pesticide reduction of 75%. Additionally, the vegetables met the quality standards for green food.

Table 4. Control effects of soil treatment on the striped flea beetle

Soil treatment	Decline rate of beetle (%)			Deterrent effect (%)
	5d	15d	20d	
Tobacco	94.12	68.57	73.08	79.78
EM fertilizer	76.47	57.14	19.23	47.55
NH_4HCO_3	82.35	37.14	11.54	42.16
Lime	29.41	22.86	12.76	18.38
Phoxim	88.24	60.00	19.23	57.11

5. Integrated Development of a Sustainable Pest Control System

On the basis of the aforementioned efforts to develop key technologies, we integrated them and developed a sustainable control system for the major pests of cruciferous vegetables. This system prioritizes protecting both field biodiversity and the biological control activities of natural enemies; its core technologies involve habitat management and biological control. Subsequently, taking the different seasonal occurrence patterns of the main pests into account, our system integrates various new techniques in pest behavioral modulation, disorienting prevention, pesticide reduction and chemical control and organizes them into three subsystems (You and Hou, 2004; Liu and Hou, 2004). First, the dominant pests in spring (March to June) are *P. striolata* and *P. xylostella*, which are controlled by pathogenic nematodes, sex attractants and vegetable protective agents (Figure 14). Second, the dominant species in summer (June to September) are *Spodoptera* spp.(e.g., *S. litura*), which are suppressed by insect viruses, sex attractants and vegetable protective agents (Figure 15).

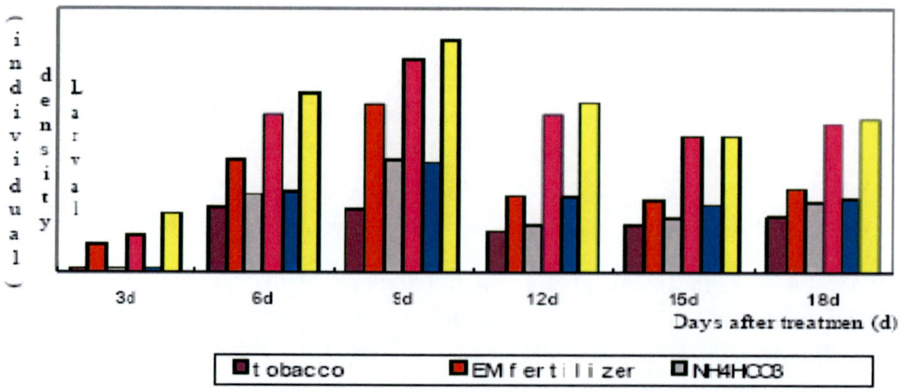

Figure 14. Effects of soil treatment on the larval dynamics of the striped flea beetle.

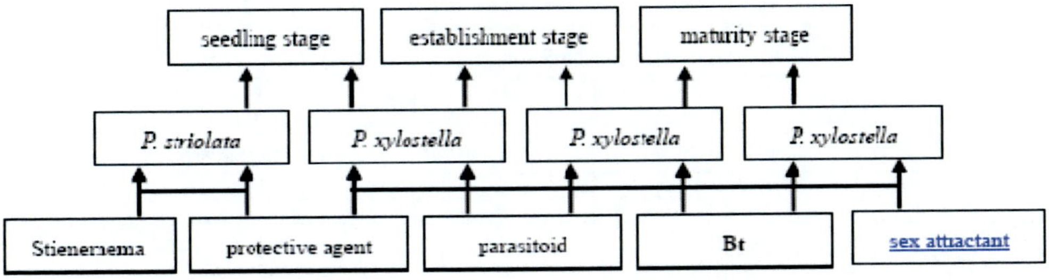

Batch	Control effect on *P. striolata* (I)	Control effect on *P. xylostella* (I)	Seedling protecting effect (%)	Production protecting effect (%)
1st batch	0.3861	0.8432	88.4	82.6
2nd batch	0.3412	0.7935	90.2	86.5

Figure 15. Sketch map of the sustainable control system for major insect pests in cruciferous vegetable in spring and its control effect.

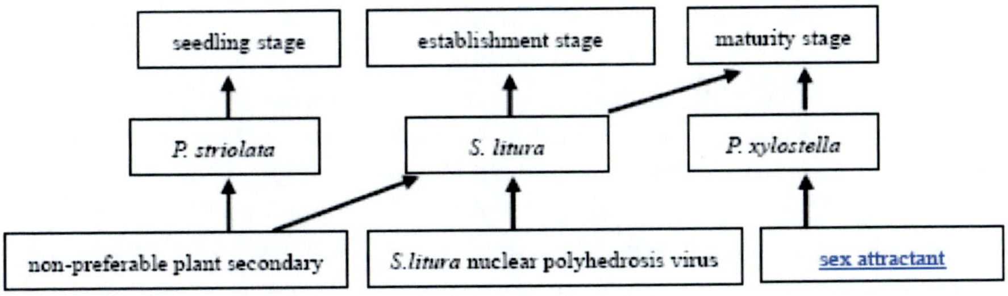

Batch	Control effect on *Prodenia litura* (I))	Seedling protecting effect (%)	Production protecting effect (%)
1st batch	0.6317	90.34	86.31
2nd batch	0.5841	91.76	87.42

Figure 16. Sketch map of the sustainable control system for major insect pests in cruciferous vegetable in summer and its control effect.

Third, the dominant species in fall (September to December) are *P. striolata* and *P. xylostella*, which are inhibited by soil treatments, natural enemy release and light trapping (Figure 16). Furthermore, we formulated three local standards for pest forecasting, ecologically-based control and pesticide resistance monitoring. We also established "Production Techniques and Processes for Green Vegetables", thereby elevating the level of safe vegetable production and facilitating the production of vegetables that meet green-food quality and/or export quality standards.

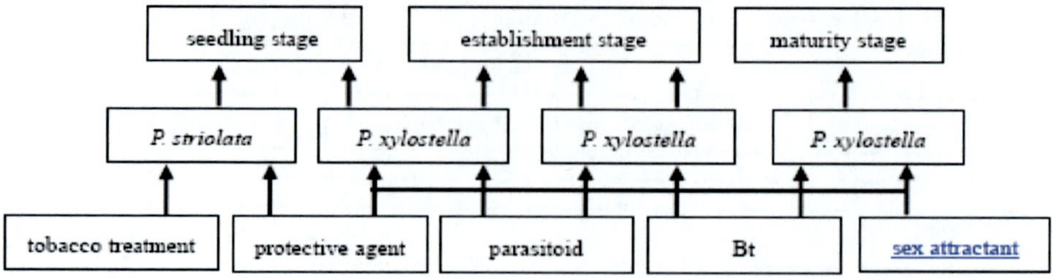

Batch	Control effect on *P. striolata*		Control effect on *P. xylostella* (I)	Seedling protecting effect (%)	Production protecting effect (%)
	Sustainable hazard index A	I			
1st batch	51.37	0.7316	0.8597	82.37	80.69
2nd batch	48.37	0.6928	0.8234	85.41	81.64

Figure 17. Sketch map of the sustainable control system for major insect pests in cruciferous vegetable in autumn and its control effect.

Meanwhile, we also developed management software that integrates safe production technologies for vegetables and process- and quality-oriented monitoring. Specifically, it covers various components in the production processes of green vegetables, including selection of a production base, farming activities, cultivation management, integrated pest control, harvesting/processing and the industrial standards and assessment procedures for green vegetables. This software applies multimedia techniques throughout the entire process of safe vegetable production and quality monitoring, thereby addressing the conflicts between production needs and expert availability (limiting the number, time and service range of experts) and revolutionizing traditional methods of promoting plant protection technologies.

CONCLUSION

Cruciferous vegetables are one of the important food crops, and widely grown in China. The crops are heavily damaged by insect pests that often causehuge losses on vegetable yield and quality.Many problems have arisen due to the overuse or misuse of chemical pesticides for pest control, which have largely influenced the food safety, environmental quality, and sustainable production of vegetables.

To meet the challenges of chemically-based pest management and the demand of healthy vegetables, since the 1990s we started to develop and implement an integrated pest management (IPM) program to incorporate various environmentally benign approaches, including habitat management, conservation biological control and behavior regulation, into an operational system.The system was designed as a flexible framework to positively favor environments for natural enemies and vegetable production. The IPM program has been extensively used to effectively control the major insect pests in cruciferous crops in the southern provinces of China, and well proved to be ecologically sound, economically feasible, environmentally acceptable, and practically applicable.The integrated management of vegetable pests is still in progress with the development of ecological entomology and bio-technology. We will continue to work in collaboration with national and international scientists engaged in this field to make pest management more effective, vegetable production more sustainable, as well as being increasingly compatible with environmental protection and natural conservation.

ACKNOWLEDGEMENTS

This work was supported by the National Key Project of Fundamental Scientific Research in China ("973" Programs, No. 2011CB100404), and the projects of the National Natural Science Foundation of China (No. 30871649, 30970528, and 30971925).

REFERENCES

Amano, K. 1984. Host preference of the yellow striped flea beetle, *Phyllotretastriolata* Fab. *Annual Report of the Society of Plant Protection of North Japan*,, 35: 132-135.

Cai, H.J., Li, Z.S.and You, M.S. 2007. Impact of habitat diversification on arthropod communities: a study in the fields of Chinese cabbage, *Brassica chinesis*. *Journal of insect science*, 14: 241-249.

Cai, H.J. and You, M.S. 2007. Effects of garlic-Chinese cabbage intercropping systems on the guilds of arthropod communities in vegetable fields. *Entomological Jouraal of East China*, 16: 1-7. (in Chinese).

Cai, H.J., You, M.S.and Lin, C. 2010. Effects of intercropping systems on community composition and diversity of predatory arthropods in vegetable fields. *Acta Ecologica Sinica*, 30: 190-195.

Cai, H.J., You, M.S., Li, S.Y., Ryall, K. and Wang, H.Y. 2011. Physiological response of Chinese cabbage to intercropping systems. *Agronomy Journal*,103, 1-6.

Chen, Z.Q., Chen, A.D., Miao, S., Luo, K.J. and Jiang, Y. 2001a. Progress in the research of the parasitoids species of *Plutella xylostella*(L.) and their introduction and utilization in China. *Journal of Yunnan Agricultural University*, 16: 308-312. (in Chinese).

Chen, Z.Q., Miao, S., Chen, A.D., Luo, and K.J. 2001. Research on the technological process of mass-rearing *Dladegma semiclausum* in laboratory. *Natural Enemies of Insects*, 23: 145-148. (in Chinese).

Chen, Z.Q., Miao, S.,Yang, C.X., Luo, K.J., Chen, A.D. and Mu, W.D. 2003.Introduction of a larval parasitoid,*Diadegma semiclausum* Hellen, and evaluation of its potency ofcontrolling *Plutella xylostella*L.*Plant Protection*, 29: 22-24. (in Chinese).

Chen, Z.Q., Miao, S.,Yang, C.X. and Luo, K.J. 2000. Introduction, release and colonization of a larval parasitoid of *Plutella xylostella*L.. *Yunnan Agricultural Science and Technology*, 6: 14-15. (in Chinese)

Deng, Y.P., Wang, Z.G., Jiang, J.X. and Du, J.W. 2007. Field behavioral responses of the male diamondback moth, *Plutella xylostella* to different components, ratios and dosages of synthetic sex attractant in China. *Journal of Zhejiang University (Agric. and Life Sci.)*, 33: 514-518.

Fu, J.W., Chen, X.L. and You, M.S. 2008. Population diferentiation of the striped flea beetle *Phyllotreta striolata*: RAPD analysis. *Chinese Journal of Ecology*, 27: 2141-2145. (in Chinese)

Fu, J.W., Li, J.Y., Qiu, L.M., Lin, Z.Y. and You, M.S. The regional diversity of susceptibility of the striped flea beetle (SFB), *Phyllotreta striolata* (Fabricius), to insecticides in Fujian Provinc. *Journal of Fujian Agriculture and Forestry University(Natural Science Edition)*, 35, 235-238. (in Chinese)

Fu, J.W., Lin, Z.Y., Li Z.S., Hou, Y.M. and You, M.S. 2004. Trapping effect of yellow sticky board on the insect pests of vegetables and the application to the monitoring population of the striped flea beetle *Phyllotreta striolata* (F.). *Journal of Fujian Agriculture and Forestry University(Natural Science Edition)*, 33: 438-440. (in Chinese)

Fu, J.W., Xu, D.M., Wu, W. and You, M.S. 2005. Preference of different vegetable insect pests to color. *Chinese Bulletin of Entomology*, 42: 532-533. (in Chinese)

Fu, J.W. and You, M.S. 2004. Effects of host plants on the activity of enzymes related to pesticide resistance of the striped flea beetle, *Phyllotreta striolata* (Coleoptera: Chrysomelidae). *Journal of Fujian Agriculture and Forestry University(Natural Science Edition)*, 33: 153-157. (in Chinese).

He, Y.R. 1998. Studies on the population control of the diamondback moth, *Plutella xylostella*(L.), with trichogramma and other parasitoids. South China Agricultural University Press, Guangzhou. (in Chinese)

He, Y.X., Wang, C.F., Chen, F., Yang, X.J. and Weng, Q.Y. 2003. Effect of insecticides on esterase activity in the beet armyworm (*Spodoptera exigua*). *Acta Agriculturae Universitatis Jiangxiensis*, 25: 896-899. (in Chinese)

Hou, Y.M., You, M.S., Pang, X.F. and Liang, G.W. 2000a. Structure and quantity dynamic of arthropod communities in vegetable fields. *Journal of Fujian Agriculture University*, 29: 323-328. (in Chinese).

Hou, Y.M., Peng, X.F., Liang, G.W. and Chen, S.P. 2000b. Study on the control effect of the soil treatment on the population of the striped flea beetle [*Plyllotreta striolata* (F.)]. *Journal South China Agricultural University*, 21: 21-24. (in Chinese)

Hou, Y.M., Pang, X.F. and Liang, G.W. 2000c. Appliedtechnologyof synthetic sex pheromonesin vegetable fields to control the population of the diamondback moth, *Plutella xylostella* L. *Natural Enemies of Insects*, 22: 111-115. (in Chinese)

Hou, Y.M., Pang, X.F. and Liang, G.W. 2001a. On the partial application of steinernema carpocapsae strain A24 against the striped flea beetle phyllotreta striolata. *Acta Phytophylacica Sinica*, 28: 152-156. (in Chinese)

Hou, Y.M., You, M.S., Pang, X.F. and Liang, G.W. 2001b. Application technology of entomopathogenic nematodes to control the striped flea beetle in vegetable fields. *Journal of Fujian Agricultural University*, 30: 67-71. (in Chinese).

Hou, Y.M., Pang, X.F., Liang, G.W. and You, M.S. 2001c. Effect of chemical insecticides on the diversity of arthropods invegetable fields. *Acta Ecologica Sinica*, 21: 1262-1268. (in Chinese)

Hou, Y.M., Pang, X.F., Liang, G.W. and You, M.S. 2001d. Control effect of *Plutella xylostella* with synthetic sex pheromone. *Chinese Journal of Biological Control*, 17: 121-125. (in Chinese)

Hou, Y.M. 2001. Control mechanism of secondary metabolites of non-host plants on major pests of vegetables. Fujian Agriculture and Forestry University Press, Fuzhou. (in Chinese)

Hou, Y.M., Pang, X.F. and Liang, G.W. 2002. Effects of azadirachtin against the diamondback moth, *Plutella xylostella. Acta Entomologica Sinica*, 45: 47-52.(in Chinese)

Hou, Y.M., Pang, X.F., Liang, G.W. and You, M.S. 2003. Evaluation of azadirachtin against the striped flea beetle, *Phyllotreta striolata* (F.). *Chinese Journal of Applied Ecology*, 14: 959-962. (in Chinese)

Jiang, D.H., Deng, R.Q., Pang, Y. and Long, Q.X. 1997. The new bacillus thuringiensis isolates highly toxic*Prodenia litura* larvae and their characterization.*Microbiology*, 24: 262-265. (in Chinese)

Jiang, J.X., Zeng, A.P., Ji, X.Y. and Jiang, Z.R. 2005. Vertical transmission of *Spodoptera exigua* nuclear polyhedrosis virus in the beetarmyworm, *Spodotera exigua.Acta Entomologica Sinic*, 48: 922-927. (in Chinese)

Jiang, J.X., Jiang, Z.R. and Lei, R.H. 2004. Cooperative effect of *Spodoptera litura* nuclear polyhedrosis virus with a parasite wasp, *Microplitis sp.*on the *S. litura* larvae. *Chinese Journal of Applied Ecology*, 15: 303-307. (in Chinese)

Jiang, J.X., Zeng, A.P., Ji, X.Y. and Wan, N.F. 2011. Combined effect of nucleopoly-hedrovirus and microplitispallidipes for the control of the beet armyworm, *Spodopteraexigua. Pest Management Science*, 67: 705-713.

Joshi, B.G., Sitaramaiah, S.and Ramaprasad, G. 1982. Field observations on the impact of the egg parasite *Telenomusremus*(Hymenoptera: Scelionidae) on the tobacco caterpillar, *Spodopteralitura* (Lepidoptera: Noctuidae) in tobacco nurseries in Andhra Pradesh, India. *Entomophaga*, 27: 331-334.

Lai, R.Q. and You, M.S. 2005. Anti-feeding effect of the extracts from non-preferable plants onadults of the striped flea beetle [*Phyllotreta striolata* (F.)]. *Plant Protection*, 31: 37-40. (in Chinese)

Liu, B., Cai, Y.C. and Guan, X. (2004) *Theory and practice of food safety*. Haifeng Press, Fuzhou. pp. 232-235. (in Chinese)

Liu, X., You, M.S., Wu, M.X., Huang, B. and Huang, J.M. 1998. Construction of the natural population life table of the diamondback mothand analysis of its important factors. *Journal of Fujian Agricultural University*, 27: 177-180. (in Chinese)

Liu, X. and You, M.S. 1998. Effect of pesticides on the laboratory population of *Plutella xylostella* (L.). *Entomological Journal of East China*, 7, 103-106. (in Chinese)

Liu, X. and You, M.S. 2003. Construction and important factors analysis of natural life table of the diamonthback moth *Plutella xylostella* underpesticides treatment. *Chinese Journal of Applied Ecology*, 14: 1395-1397. (in Chinese)

Liu, B., Cai, Y.C. and Guan, X. 2004. *Theory and practice of food safety*. Haifeng Press, Fuzhou. pp. 350-355. (in Chinese)

Liu, Y., You, M.S. and Hou, Y.M. 2005. A new method of rearing the laboratory population of the striped flea beetle, *Phyllotreta striolata. Chinese Bulletin of Entomology*, 42: 578-581. (in Chinese)

Liu, Y. and You, M.S.2008. The life table of the experimental population of the striped flea beetle. *Journal of Fujian Agriculture and Forestry University(Natural Science Edition)*, 37: 27-33. (in Chinese)

Lü, L.H. 1998. Role of *Plutella xylostella* granulosis virus in ecological control of the diamondback moth, *Plutella xylostella.* South China Agricultural University Press, Guangzhou. (in Chinese)

Lu, X.S., Weng Q.Y., Wang, C.F., Yang, X.J. and He, Y.X. 2003. Studies on active regularity of adult *Bemisia tabaci* by using yellow sticky traps. *Fujian Journal of Agricultural Sciences*, 18: 233-235. (in Chinese)

Lü, Y.B. and Liu, S.S. 2004. Effects of plant responses induced by exogenous jasmonic acid on host-selection behavior of *Cotesia plutellae* (Hymenoptera: Braconidae). *Acta Entomologica Sinia*, 47: 206-212. (in Chinese)

Lü, Y.B., Liu, S.S., Liu, Y.Q., Furlong, M.J. and Zalucki, M.P. 2004. Contrary effects of jasmonate treatment of two closely related plant species on the attraction of and oviposition by a specialist herbivore. *Ecology Letter*, 7: 337-345.

Lü, Y.B. and Liu, S.S. 2005. Effects of exogenous jasmonic acid-induced plant responses on the development and growth of *Plutella xylostella. Chinese Journal of Applied Ecology*, 16: 193-195. (in Chinese)

Si, S.Y., Liu, X.M., Wang, Y. and Wu, R.F. 2005. Occurrence and integrated pest management of the beet armyworm, *Spodoptera exigua*in Wuhan. *Journal of Changjiang Vegetables*, 8: 38-39. (in Chinese)

Si, S.Y., Wu, R.F., Liu, X.M. and. Zhou, F. 2001. Current Situation and management strategies of insecticide resistance of the diamondback moth and beet armyworm. *Journal of Changjiang Vegetables*, 1: 6-8. (in Chinese)

Talekar, N.S., and Sheton, A.M. 1993. Biology ecology and management of the diamondback moth. *Annual Review of Entomology*, 38: 275-301.

Wan, N.F., Jiang, J.X., Ji, X.Y. and Yang, Y.J. 2008. Preliminary report on the effect of frequency oscillation lampson trapping insect pests and the insect pests'rhythm of dashingat lamps in protected horticultural fields. *Acta Agriculturae Shanghai*, 24: 65-68. (in Chinese)

Wang, C.L., Wu, S.W., Yang, Y.H. and Wu, Y.D. 2006. Field-evolved resistance to Bt δ-endotoxins and Bt formulation in *Plutella xylostella* from the southeastern coast region of China. *Acta Entomologica Sinica*, 49: 70-73. (in Chinese)

Wang, X.R. and Li, S.C. 1994. Activity of the entomoparasitic nematode *Heterorhabditis sp.* (Taishan No. 1) tested against *Spodoptera litura* (F.). *Journal of Zhongkai University of Agriculture and Technology*, 7: 28-32. (in Chinese)

Wei, H., Hou, Y.M., Yang, G., Fu, J.W. and You, M.S. 2005. Evaluation of non-host plant ethanol extracts against the *Plutella xylostella* population. *Chinese Journal of Applied Ecology*, 16: 1086-1089. (in Chinese)

Wei, H., Hou, Y.M., Yang, G. and You, M.S. 2004. Repellent and anti-feedant effect of secondary metabolites of non-host plants on *Plutella xylostella.Chinese Journal of Applied Ecology*, 15: 473-476. (in Chinese)

Wu, M.X. and You, M.S. 2001. Investigations on natural enemies of the diamondback moth in the Suburbs of Fuzhou. *Entomological Journal of East China*, 10: 25-28. (in Chinese)

Wykie, H.G. 1984. Oviposition and survival of three Nearctic euphorine in cruciferinfesting flea beetles. *Can Entomol.*, 116: 1-4.

Xu, Q.Y. and You, M.S. 1999. Structure and dynamics of insect communities in crucifer. *Journal of Fujian Agricultural University*, 28: 175-180. (in Chinese)

Yan, Z.M., Hou, Y.M. and Luo, W.C. 2005. Bio-activities of the extracts from *Lantana camara* on the adult of striped flea beetles, *Phyllotreta striolata. Chinese Bulletin of Entomology*, 42: 664-66. (in Chinese)

Yang, G., Xu, Q.Y. and You, M.S. 2004b. The change of activities of protective enzymes in Chinese cabbage infested by the diamondback moth, *Plutella xylostella. Entomological Journal of East China*, 13: 48-54. (in Chinese)

Yang, G., You, M.S. and Wei, H. 2004a. Component and content changes of volatiles from Chinese cabbage damaged by *Plutellaxylostella. Chinese Journal of Applied Ecology*, 15: 2157-2160. (in Chinese)

Yang, G., Wang, D.F., Dong, Z.Q., Wang, Q.L., Wang-PruskiGefu, and You, M.S. 2011. Characterization of a myrosinasecDNA from *Brassica parachinensis* and its defense role against *Plutellaxylostella* after suppression. *Insect Science*, (accepted).

You, M.S.and Hou, Y.M.2004. Ecological control system of the diamondback moth in cruciferous vegetable fields. IN: Proceedings of the 15th International Plant Protection Congress. pp. 11-16. Beijing, China.

You, M.S., Hou, Y.M. and Yang, G. 2003. *Control of diamondback moth population system.* Fujian Science and Technology Press, Fuzhou.

You, M.S., Liu, Y.F. and Hou, Y.M. 2004. Biodiversity and integrated pest management in agroecosystems. *Acta Ecologica Sinica*, 24: 117-122. (in Chinese)

You, M.S. and Xu, Q.Y. 2000. Species Composition, richness and diversity of insect communities in cruciferous fields in Fouzhou's suburb.*Journal of Fujian Agricultural University*, 29: 444-452.

You, M.S. and Yang, G. 2001. Physiological stress reaction of Chinese cabbage, *Brassica chinensis*, infested by the diamondback moth, *Plutellaxylostella.EntomologiaSinica*, 8: 131-140.

Zhang G.Z. and You, M.S. 2009. Measurement of the active ingredient of *Macleya cordata* and its bioactivity against insects. *Journal of Anhui Agricultural Universit*, 36: 18-21. (in Chinese)

Zhang G.Z. and You, M.S. 2008. Study on the Insecticidal Action of*Macleaya cordata. Journal of Anhui Agricultural Sciences*, 36: 7312-7313. (in Chinese)

Zhang, M.X. 1998. Studies on the population dynamics of the striped flea beetle,*Phyllotreta striolata*(Fabricius) and its control. South China Agricultural University Press, Guangzhou. (in Chinese)

Zhang, M.L. 1997. Effect of 14 insecticides on adults, larvae, eggs, and pupae of trichogramma confusum. *Natural Enemies of Insects*, 19: 11-14. (in Chinese)

Zhao, X.Y. and Hou, Y.M. 2006. Bioactivity of the essential oil from dragon juniper against the diamondback moth(*Plutella xylostella*). *Chinese Bulletin of Entomology*, 43: 57-60. (in Chinese)

Zheng, L.Z., Fu, J.W., Chen, X.L., Zhong, X.L. and You, M.S. 2009. Mechanism on the susceptibility of the striped flea beetle, Phyllotreta striolata to chlorpyrifos.*Chinese Bulletin of Entomology*, 46: 256-259. (in Chinese)

Zhou, J.W., He, Y.X. and Weng, Q.Y. 2008. Application and research of insect light traps in China. *Entomological Journal of East China*, 17: 76-80. (in Chinese)

Zhou, L.L., Si, S.Y., Wang, Z.X., Wang, Y. and Liu X.M. 2009. Biochemical mechanisms of the beet armyworm's (*Spodoptera exigua*)resistanceto tebufenozide.*Acta Entomologica Sinica*, 52: 386-394. (in Chinese)

Zhou, X.M., Jiang, J.X., Wan N.F. and Zhu Y.F. 2009. Effects of vertical transmission of virus in *Spotoptera litura* fabricius adults on its progeny. *Journal of Anhui Agricultural Sciences*, 37: 15897-15898. (in Chinese)

Zhu, S.X., Si, S.Y., Zhou, F. and Liu, X.M. 1996. Analysis on the pesticide-resistant character of the diamondback moth (*Plutella xylostella*) and field monitoring. *Entomological Knowledge*, 33, 82-85. (in Chinese)

Zhu, Y.F., Wan, N.F., Ji, X.Y., Chen, X.Q. and Jiang, J.X. 2007. Virulence determination of 7 pesitcides to *Prodenia litura* and *Spodoptera exigua*. *Journal of Changjiang Vegetables*, 2: 60-61. (in Chinese).

Zhou, F. and Si, S.Y. 1996. Outddoreffects of Bt-basedinsecticides onthe diamondback moth. *Journal of Changjiang Vegetables*, 9: 13-15. (in Chinese).

In: Vegetable Consumption and Health: New Research
Editors: Claudia Wilson and Melinda Morree
ISBN: 978-1-62100-941-2

Chapter 5

AVAILABILITY AND UTILIZATION OF TRADITIONAL VEGETABLES: A CASE STUDY OF RURAL XHOSA HOUSEHOLDS

T. P. Dweba[1,*] and M. A. Mearns[2,†]

[1]Department of Agriculture, Animal Health and Human Ecology, University of South Africa, P.O. Box 392, Unisa, South Africa

[2]Department of Information and Knowledge Management, University of Johannesburg, PO Box 524, Auckland Park, South Africa

ABSTRACT

Micronutrient deficiency is a major challenge in resource poor households of South Africa. While traditional vegetables have been identified as one of the strategies to alleviate micronutrient deficiency in such households, research has shown a decline in the use of traditional vegetables in favour of introduced vegetables. Traditional vegetables, unlike introduced vegetables, can survive poor soil, require less agricultural inputs and resources during production and are often available at times when introduced vegetables are scarce. Knowledge about traditional vegetables is vanishing due to the decline in traditional vegetable use. Since documentation of traditional vegetables is scarce, elderly people remain the most valuable source of knowledge. Due to a general reluctance of the youth to gain knowledge associated with the utilisation of traditional vegetables, the fear exist that valuable indigenous knowledge on traditional vegetables might disappear completely from society.

Research was conducted to determine the availability of traditional vegetables at eMantlaneni village close to Lusikisiki in the Eastern Cape Province of South Africa. The extent of traditional vegetable use was determined and the collection, storage, preservation and cooking practices of traditional vegetables were documented. The larger significance of the research not only lies in the documentation of the associated indigenous knowledge that is in danger of being lost, but also in establishing utilisation patterns that can be used to compare regional variations in collection,

* mbombtp@unisa.ac.za (T.P. Dweba).
† Corresponding author: M.A. Mearns. Tel: +2711 559 4700, Fax +2711 559 2822, mearnsm@uj.ac.za.

storage, cooking and preservation practices. The study envisioned that more knowledge about traditional vegetables could improve food diversity which will translate to the improvement of nutritional status of resource poor households.

The research was limited to a single case study, documenting the practices of one South African cultural grouping (Xhosa cultural practices). The study could also not include the nutritional value of the traditional vegetables, although this has been identified as need for further research. Main findings of the research showed that thirty three (33) traditional vegetables were identified and their collection, storage, preservation and cooking practices were described. Already accessibility to some traditional vegetables poses a problem due to women having to travel long distances to gather these scarce traditional vegetables. The study concluded that the suitability of traditional vegetables rests on their benefits of being readily available, low agricultural input and reported nutritional value. Because of these benefits traditional vegetables can contribute towards food diversity and food security, however, the benefits can only be reaped if the indigenous knowledge associated with traditional vegetables is available.

1. Introduction

In this chapter the term traditional vegetables is used to define vegetables that form part of local cuisine and have originated in a particular area as well as those that are considered local due to their physiologically adaptation to local conditions after being introduced (Nesamvuni, 2000, p.14; Laker, 2007, p.311). The aptness of traditional vegetables lies in the plant's excellent survival attributes, and the reported outstanding nutritional qualities as a food source. Unlike other vegetable counterparts, traditional vegetables are readily available and or are grown with minimal or no agricultural inputs. They are harvested from both cultivated lands and uncultivated lands. Traditional vegetables require less resources, chemical fertilizers and pesticides during production since they are well suited to local conditions. Traditional vegetables endure poor soils and harsh climatic conditions such as drought and unreliable rainfall. They are often available when other introduced vegetables such as tomato and cabbage are not (Lephole, 2004; Modi, Modi, & Hendricks, 2006; Nesamvuni, 2000; Van Vuuren, 2006). Furthermore, traditional vegetables are believed to have considerable amounts of nutrients and minerals such as vitamin A, vitamin C, folic acid, iron, manganese, calcium and zinc (Uusiku, Oelofse, Duodu, Bester & Faber, 2010; Van Vuuren, 2006, p.24; Lephole, 2004, p.67; Nesamvuni, 2000, p.96).

Knowledge about traditional vegetables forms part of indigenous knowledge systems. This knowledge is passed from one generation to the other as part of indigenous knowledge in the community and is often not documented. As a result knowledge on traditional vegetables like other types of indigenous knowledge system is lost and their utilisation is diminishing. The reduced consumption of traditional vegetables is due to factors such as introduction of new vegetables, historical policies, stigma, habitat loss and changes in lifestyle (Dweba & Mearns, 2011, pp. 2-3). Furthermore, traditional vegetables are often labelled as 'famine foods' and indigenous knowledge as 'backward knowledge' by communities. The negative labels given to traditional vegetables have led to a further decline in consumption of traditional vegetables even in rural areas (Vorster, Jansen van Rensburg, Van Zijil & Venter, 2007a). This reduced consumption of traditional vegetables has dire consequences on diet diversity of resource poor communities who have limited access to other vegetables (Flyman & Afoloyan, 2006, pp. 492-497).

The perceived loss of traditional vegetable knowledge is further augmented by younger women's (women aged between 20 and 30 years) reluctance to learn about traditional vegetables due to the stigma that is attached to these vegetables. The impact of the stigma is evident in the younger women's preference of introduced vegetables over traditional vegetables (Vorster, *et al.,* 2007a, p.3). Habitually the younger generation would play a major role in preserving traditional knowledge as it is undocumented but passed from the older generation to the younger. However, the lack of enthusiasm amongst the younger generation to learn about traditional vegetables could lead to complete erosion of traditional vegetable knowledge. This fear of loss of knowledge has incited the need to conserve traditional vegetable knowledge through documentation and gene-banks (Vorster, Jansen Van Rensburg, Van Zijil & Venter, 2007b, p.11).

Research was therefore undertaken to document the availability of traditional vegetables at a rural village in South Africa. The utilisation patterns and potential future use of traditional vegetables was investigated. Due to the high prevalence of micronutrient deficiencies in South Africa it is not surprising that a number of strategies such as supplementation, food fortification, bio fortification, food diversification and public health programs have been proposed to be used in combination (Faber, Laurie & Venter, 2006, p.14). Use of food-based strategies as part of food diversification to alleviate micronutrient deficiency is a point of departure for this chapter and traditional vegetables could provide an exceptional alternative source of minerals and nutrients, especially amongst resource poor communities, to improve their diet diversity and nutritional status.

2. Background of the Study Area and Justification

The Eastern Cape Province is located in the south-eastern part of South Africa and the research was conducted in a village which is situated in the north-east corner of the Province. The province is the third most populous province in South Africa and the second poorest province in the country. According to Aphane, Chadha & Olouch (2003, p.9) the Eastern Cape Province is amongst four provinces that have the highest incidences of food insecurity and malnutrition in South Africa. There are six district municipalities in this province namely: Alfred Nzo, Amatole, Cacadu, Chris Hani, OR Tambo and Ukhahlamba. eMantlaneni village is located near the town of Lusikisiki, within the Qaukeni Local Municipality which is occupied by Xhosa speaking people. Qaukeni Local Municipality falls under OR Tambo district municipality. This district municipality is mostly rural with a population of about 1.7 million people. It is characterized by high levels of unemployment, and large pockets of poverty. The OR Tambo district municipality has the poorest access to basic services of all the district municipalities and this is particularly essential because it has a direct impact on the quality of life of inhabitants. The Lusikisiki town and surrounding areas receives medium-low rainfall and is characterized by poor soils (Eastern Cape Provincial Government, 2003, pp.18-57).

This therefore means there is an urgent need to explore various strategies to address food insecurity and malnutrition not just in the area where the study was conducted but in other areas that have similar climatic and ecological characteristics. Food diversification has been proposed by many researchers as one of the strategies to improve nutritional intake mainly because of its long-term sustainability and affordability. This strategy focuses on increasing availability and accessibility of nutrient-rich foods with the expectation to increase their consumption. Due to the high prices of animal sources which are often out of economic reach for resource poor communities, foods of plant origin are highly recommended (Aphane et al., 2003, p.9; Faber et al., 2006, p14). Given the characteristics of traditional vegetables, it is therefore justified to assume that traditional vegetables would make a reasonable contribution towards alleviating food insecurity in the study area and areas with similar characteristics. Traditional vegetables can potentially provide these people with direct access to vitamin and mineral rich foods, even those that are unable to grow their home gardens due to limited resources.

Furthermore, the advocacy of the use of traditional vegetables is further protracted by the locale where the study was conducted. Like many rural areas in the Eastern Cape, the area where the study was conducted is faced with serious challenges regarding accessibility of markets due to distance to markets, poor road conditions, infrastructure, as well as poor and costly public transport. This inaccessibility of fresh produce could have a negative effect on diet diversity and nutrition for those households that do not grow their own fresh produce. Dweba & Mearns (2011, p. 2); Vorster et al. (2007a, p.7) are of the opinion that geographical isolation and poor road conditions of the area has a direct effect on the difficulty to access markets and inaccessibility of fresh vegetables. Easy access and frequency of access to fresh vegetables is highly essential to ensure their regular inclusion in the diet as they are highly perishable.

In addition to the geographical isolation of the area, the other contributing factor is the socio-economic status of the people concerned. Socio-economic data plays a major role in determining food choices. Inadequate financial resources limit the amount of money that is available to be spent on food thus causing people to opt for cheaper alternatives. The buying power not only limits the kind of foods that is bought but the frequency as well (Viljoen, Botha & Boonzaaier, 2005, p.56). Research findings from the study conducted at eMantlaneni village revealed that most of the respondents had lower incomes and belong to significant large households (on average more than six members per household). In addition to that, these large households had fewer income earners, a factor that could stretch their financial resources even further. These statistics corresponds with the literature, namely that the region where the study was conducted has the highest number of persons (82%) living in poverty (Eastern Cape Provincial Government, 2003, pp.18-57; Ingquza Hill Local Municipality, 2007, pp.33-34; Alemu, 2010, pp.1-23). This supports the need for researching the current and potentially the future use of traditional vegetables as a cheaper alternative food source. Lephole, (2004); Modi et al., (2006); Nesamvuni, (2000); Van de Heever, (1995) and Van Vuuren (2006) arrived at a similar conclusion, accentuating the role that could be played by traditional vegetables on diet diversity and nutritional status of low income earners.

As to be expected from the reported reluctance of the younger generation to learn about and utilise traditional vegetables a negative attitudes towards the use of traditional vegetables were discovered. According to previous studies similar lower levels of acceptance for traditional vegetables were found (Keller, Mndiga & Maass, 2006, pp.400-413; Vorster *et al.*, 2007a, p.6; Modi *et al.*, 2006;). Apart from the stigma associated with traditional vegetables and changes in lifestyle, this could be associated to education and urbanisation that is instilling new values and attitudes among youth at the expense of their cultural norms (Shava, 2000, pp.34-35). Furthermore, the decline in utilisation could be further attributed to the youth finding preparation methods of traditional vegetables as boring (Vorster, et al., 2007b, p.9). In addition, one should never underestimate the role played by status associated with certain foods and peer pressure when making food choices. Especially youth would choose only what is believed to endow greater social standing amongst their peers, therefore the reported negative labels contribute to further rejection of traditional vegetables (Kittler & Sucher, 2000, pp.3-4). Reduced consumption of traditional vegetables by the youth is a major concern as it forecasts a bleak future for the consumption of traditional vegetables and is the first sign leading towards loss of use and knowledge about traditional vegetables (Keller et al., 2006, pp.10-411). To confirm these claims the research at eMantlaneni village consisted of interviews and focus group discussions of both older and younger women to document associated indigenous knowledge and determine attitudes and perceptions towards traditional vegetables.

3. Description of the Research at Emantlaneni

The consumption of traditional vegetables is decreasing even in the rural areas of South Africa, in favour of introduced vegetables. The neglect by both policy makers and researchers has led to the scarcity of information on traditional vegetables (Aphane *et al.*, 2003; Van Rensberg *et al.*, 2007b, pp.317-324). Since documentation on traditional vegetables is scarce, elderly people remain the most valuable sources of information. The fear exists that if nothing is done to preserve valuable information on traditional vegetables this information may soon disappear from society, because the youth are generally reluctant to gain such knowledge (Vorster *et al.*, 2007b).

The study was based on the social systems theory suggested by Babbie (2008, pp.36-39); a philosophical paradigm which views the community as a social system that is made up of parts, each of which contributes to the functioning of the whole. The research paradigm that was followed used mixed methods combining the collection of qualitative data and quantitative data in an attempt to offset the weaknesses inherent within one method with the strengths of the other method. The study comprised two samples, namely 16 young women and 38 elderly women. The first study sample of 16 young women from the village was divided into two focus groups, eight in each. Selection criteria for this group were women between the ages of 20 to 30 years of age and the aim was to determine their attitudes towards traditional vegetable use. The younger women selected randomly were included in the study as a measure to determine the potential future use of traditional vegetables based on the attitudes of the younger women towards traditional vegetables. The knowledge of younger women regarding traditional vegetables is therefore a measure of indigenous knowledge sharing that has taken place from the older generation to the younger generation. Their attitudes towards traditional vegetables are a measure of potential and possible future indigenous knowledge sharing regarding traditional vegetables to the next generation of users.

The second sample which comprised of 38 elderly women was selected to document knowledge about the availability and utilization techniques of traditional vegetables in the Xhosa households of the demarcated study area, using a semi-structured questionnaire. These women were selected using snowball sampling. The selection criteria for inclusion in the study group were elderly women aged 50 and above. The reason for this selection criterion was the fact that literature has indicated that elderly women are the main users of traditional vegetables (Nesamvuni, 2000, p.4; Odhav et al.,2007,p.430; Modi et al., 2006,p.9; Lephole, 2004,p.80). Therefore in this study, elderly women as custodians of indigenous knowledge on traditional vegetables were included as the main sources of information on the current usage, availability, collection, storage and cooking practices of traditional vegetables. The data collection through an interview administered questionnaire was followed by a focus group discussion with eight elderly women who were randomly selected from the respondents who participated in the questionnaire to triangulate and validate the information gathered during this phase and to clarify any uncertainties that might ensue after the questionnaire phase.

Lastly, plant specimens were collected to determine the availability of traditional vegetables with the help of elderly women from the villages and taken to the South African National Biodiversity Institute (SANBI) for scientific identification. Apart from providing the scientific names of the traditional vegetables, the collection of specimens also assisted in the refinement of the list to authenticate the exact number of traditional vegetables that were available in the area, as most traditional vegetables had more than one vernacular name. Herbarium procedures for collection and transportation of specimens were followed to ensure good quality of specimens as suggested by Fish (1999, p.7). Limitations of the research included the study's confinement to a single case study, therefore practices of other villages and other cultural groups in South Africa were not documented. Furthermore, the study did not investigate the nutritional value of traditional vegetables and this has been identified as a need for further research. Furthermore the research did not include nutritional analysis of the dried vegetables and the cooked dishes to determine the actual nutrient contribution of traditional vegetables to the diets of the community and the research rests on the assumptions found in the literature that traditional vegetables are generally good sources of minerals and vitamins (Uusiku *et al.*, 2010; Van Vuuren, 2006, p.24; Lephole, 2004, p.67; Nesamvuni, 2000, p.96).

4. Lessons Learned

4.1. Availability

Physical, social and economic availability and access of food are regarded as very critical aspects of food security, as they contribute to continuous access to food at household and national levels. Individual choices are influenced to a larger extent by food that people have access to and the means that people have to acquire the food (McDonald, 2010, p.2). Due to unavailability people often adapt their diets in favour of what is available (Viljoen *et al.*, 2005, p.56). There were ±30 traditional vegetables that were available at eMantlaneni village. Although 33 vegetables were identified as traditional vegetables that are availability in this village, the availability for only 30 specimens could be confirmed from the collection for identification by the herbarium. These vegetables were then grouped in 3 categories in terms of their accessibility. The approximate distance from the households ranges between 0 and 15 km. These three categories of accessibility are clearly defined in an article by Dweba &

Mearns (2011, p.4). According to this article about eight different vegetables out of the total number of traditional that are available in the village are found within a kilometre from the households. This number of accessible traditional vegetables could make a significant contribution in food diversity and food security in the community. The traditional vegetables could provide households with direct access to vitamin and mineral rich foods, and compliment home-garden production especially during drought and famine (Aphane, et al., p. 9). Although availability of traditional vegetables was found to be highly seasonal, there were seven traditional vegetables that were available throughout the year (Dweba & Mearns, 2011, pp.4-5). The availability of these traditional vegetables all year round further strengthens the prospect from the literature that the traditional vegetables are available at times when others are not (Lephole 2004; Nesamvuni 2000; Van Vuuren2006; Modi *et al.*, 2006). Therefore when maximally exploited these traditional vegetables will not only improve food security, but could provide important sources of nutrients, vitamins and minerals.

4.2. Utilisation Patterns

Considering the number of traditional vegetables that are available in the study area, their exploitation as a food source was not impressive. Out of the total vegetables that are available in this village, 20 vegetables were used by less than 30% of the studied population (Dweba & Mearns, 2011, pp.5-6). The most popular traditional vegetables (used by more than 60% of the population) were nomdlomboyi / *amaranthus viridis*, umhlabangulo/ *bidens pilosa L.*, *uswelentaka / physalis peruviana, gcamche / obetia tenax , ububazi / laportea penduncularis subsp. penduncularis,* and *imithwane / curcubita moschatar, umsobo / solanum chenopodioides Lam,* irhwaba/ *ilhaba / sonchus oleraceus L.* It would be specifically the least used traditional vegetables that face the greatest threat of loss specifically in terms of their associated indigenous knowledge. This confirms findings from the literature that traditional vegetable utilisation is decreasing (Aphane *et al.*, 2003; Van Rensberg *et al.*, 2007a; Van Rensberg *et al.*, 2007b; Shava, 2000; Keller *et al.*, 2006). Accessibility could be the reason attributed to the decreased utilisation as found by Dweba & Mearns (2011, pp.5-6) reflecting, the traditional vegetables that are least utilised are those that were found more than 1km away from the households. Reluctance to walk long distances for gathering was mentioned as one the reasons for decreased utilisation of traditional vegetables (Keller *et al.*, 2006, p.410).

4.3. Collection, Cooking and Preservation

In this study most traditional vegetables were reported to be found in both cultivated lands and uncultivated lands. Some of the vegetables grows naturally in the gardens and in the fields amongst natural vegetation while some grow along river banks (see Table 1). Only five traditional vegetables that previously grew in natural fields only have been domesticated and this has improved accessibility and utilisation to these specific traditional vegetables. They vegetables are gcamche /Obetia tenax (N.E.Br.) Friis; uswelentaka / physalis peruviana; umsobo / solanum chenopodioides Lam; ububazi / laportea penduncularis subsp. Penduncularis and iguzu/ beruala thunbergii. All these vegetables except for iguzu / beruala thunbergii were consumed by more than 60% of the respondents.

Table 1. Place where the traditional vegetables are harvested

Name of traditional vegetable	Botanical name	Cultivated lands	Natural fields	River banks
1. Gcamche	Obetia tenax (N.E.Br.) Friis	××	×	
2. Nomdlomboyi	Amaranthus viridis L.	×		
3. Umhlabangulo	Bidens Pilosa L.	×		
4. Irhwaba /Ihlaba	Sonchus oleraceus L.	×	×	
5. Ububazi	Laportea penduncularis (Wedd.)Chew subsp. Penduncularis	××	×	
6. Umsobo	Solanum chenopodioides Lam	××	×	
7. Iwatane	Unknown			×
8. Imithwane	Curcubita moschata (Duch. Ex Lam) Duch. Ex Poir	×		
9.Uswelentaka	Physalis peruviana	××	×	
10. Iguzu	Beruala thunbergii (DC.)H. Wolff	××	×	
11. Uchaphazana	Momordica foetida Schumach			×
12. Isiqashomba	Erucastrum strigosum (Thunb)O.E.Schulz	×		
13. Uvel 'egoli / uvel'emampondweni	Galinsoga parviflora	×		
14. Imbuya	Amaranthus lividus L.	×	×	
15. Uqudalele	Hypochaeris radicata L.	×	×	
16. Imbikicane	Chenopodium giganteum D. Don	×		
17. Impontshani	Polycarpon tetraphyllum (L.)L.	×		
18. Nongobozana	Centalla asiatica (L.) Urb.	×	×	
19. Indlwabulele	Cotula australis (Spreng) Hook. F.	×	×	
20. Ufinywane	Stachys sp.		×	
21.Intebe	Zantedeschia aethiopica (L.)Spreng	×	×	
22. Uhlalani	Unknown		×	
23. Ucholachola	Could not be collected for identification due to unavailability.		×	
24.Intsheb'ebhokwe	Unkown.	×		
25.Jikeleza	Lactuca serriola L.		x	
26.Umdende	Rumex sagittatus Thunb.	×		
27. Itshongwe	Pachycarpus sp.		×	
28. Ubazana	Drouguetia ambigua Wedd.		×	

Name of traditional vegetable	Botanical name	Cultivated lands	Natural fields	River banks
29. Inkanga	Conyza sumatrensis (Retz.) E. Walker var. Sumatrensis	×	×	
30. Ityumbembe	Could not be collected for identification due to unavailability.		×	
31. Unabakuse	Could not be collected for identification due to unavailability	×	×	
32. Umyeyane	Could not be collected for identification due to unavailability.		×	
33. Incobancobana	Tetragonia sp	×	×	

** Indicate domesticated traditional vegetables.

The improved consumption of domesticated traditional vegetables that was observed in this study collaborates with the findings of the study by Aju & Poopola (2010, p.106), where traditional vegetable domestication (59.09%) was found to be prevalent and resulted in regular consumption thereof. However, although cultivated lands make up a large portion of the habitat where traditional vegetables can be harvested, the significance of habitat loss in the form of natural field and riverside vegetation reduction has a direct impact on the availability of traditional vegetables. This was confirmed by scarcity and unavailability of some of the traditional vegetables when they were collected for identification. The data collected in this research once again corroborate with the literature where a concern forhabitat loss has been mentioned as one of the reasons why traditional vegetables are rapidly disappearing (Keller *et al.*, 2005:407). Similarly to the previous studies (Bhat & Rubuluza 2002:95; Shava 2000:25-26; Modi *et al.*, 2006:8-9; Vorster *et al.*, 2007:6) the collection of traditional vegetables in this study mainly remains a female domain. However, a few incidences which involved boys in collecting traditional vegetables were reported. Collection is done by picking young tender leaves without uprooting the mother plant.

Cooking is part of post-harvest methods that are employed in food to improve digestibility, palatability and availability of nutrients; and increase the shelf life of the product. These methods occur at both home and commercial levels. Preferably vegetables would be best consumed fresh and raw because of high nutrient loss during cooking, however this is not always possible due to a number of reasons (Masarirambi, Mavuso, Songwe, Nkambule & Mhazo, 2010, pp.3333-3335). In green leafy vegetables for instance, cooking among other things improves bioavailability of vitamin A and iron by weakening the structural matrix that would otherwise make these nutrients unavailable for utilization by the body (Rodriguez-Amaya 2000, p. 33). In eMantlaneni village, traditional vegetable are either cooked into a relish (*known* as *ilaxa*) or porridge (known as *isigwampa*). Porridge, a traditional dish that is very popular among the elderly women is cooked by first boiling 1 or more cut traditional vegetables for ±30minutes under high temperatures. Thereafter traditional vegetables such as *uswelentaka / physalis peruviana or iguzu / beruala thunbergii* are added to the boiling vegetables to add a bitter taste to the dish. After a few minutes excess water is drained and discarded before adding home ground maize meal. The dish is then mixed using wooden spoon and left to cook for a further 5 to 10 minutes. There is evidence to suggest that mixing traditional vegetables with maize meal and eating it as one dish is an old practice among Xhosa people (Rose 1973, p.1355; Bhat & Rubuluza 2002, p.95; Vorster *et al.*, 2007a, p.6). The main reason behind this practice was to relieve monotony (Rose 1973, p.1355).

A relish was described as a mixture of one or more vegetables which are cut and cooked with water under high temperatures for at least 30 minutes. Excess water is then drained and discarded. Ingredients such as onion, oil and modern spices are added. This dish is then served as a side dish and eaten by all members of the household. Previous studies indicated that tomato, onion and groundnuts are usually added when cooking a relish. It is suggested that the addition of these ingredients, particularly groundnuts, increases energy value, vitamin C, folate and protein intake (Nesamvuni 2000, p.98; Modi *et al.*, 2006, p.9). Even though the addition of groundnuts and tomatoes was not reported in this study, ingredients such as oil, onion and spices were reported to be added in the preparation of a relish. The addition of fat is particularly highly recommended as it increases absorption of fat-soluble vitamins (Nesamvuni 2000, p.98; Modi *et al.*, 2006, p.9; Nguni & Mwila, 2007, p.16). Basically, the addition of fat in green leafy vegetables specifically enhances the absorption of vitamin A, a fat soluble vitamin found to be more abundant in green leafy vegetable dishes in a study by Nesamvuni (2000,p.98).

Boiling is the only method that is used in eMantlaneni village to cook traditional vegetables. The use of large quantities of water and draining thereof when cooking vegetables is highly discouraged as it result in nutrient loss especially water soluble vitamins (Dweba & Mearns, 2011; Masarirambi *et al.*, 2010,p.3338). Masarirambi *et al.* (2010, p.3338) suggest that nutrient loss is merely exacerbated when excess water is drained after cooking vegetables. A loss of vitamins is further accelerated by the use of large amounts of water and longer cooking periods (Den Hartog *et al.*, 2006, pp. 69-70). The lack of variety in the cooking methods used for traditional vegetables raises concerns. The use of one method of food preparation when cooking traditional vegetables leads to monotony which translates to traditional vegetables being labelled as poverty foods (Vorster, *et al.,* 2007b, p.7; Dweba & Mearns, 2011, pp.5-6).

Traditional vegetables just like other vegetables are seasonal, with vegetable glut occurring after rains. Furthermore traditional vegetables are highly perishable therefore if nothing is done, most of the produce could be lost due to rotting. Some of the preservation methods that are normally used include freezing, irradiation, drying, refrigeration and vacuum packaging that are used to prevent decomposition. However, most of these methods except for drying are inaccessible or impractical at household level either due to complexity of the process or unavailability of infrastructure such as electricity (Masarirambi et al., 2010, p.3334). As mentioned in paragraph 4.1, only seven traditional vegetables are available throughout the year leaving 23 traditional vegetables that available after rains; therefore their preservation could help to ensure food availability especially during winter and spring when food shortages are rife. Drying was found to be the only preservation method used, practised by 82% of the respondents (Dweba & Mearns, 2011, p.6). This data corresponds with findings by Vorster *et al.* (2007b.p.7) where drying was found to be the main preservation method used for traditional vegetables.

The leaves are harvested and under direct sunlight without blanching, are placed on reed or plastic mats that are put on flat surfaces. This drying process however differs from one that is described in the literature. For example in the northern parts of South Africa, in Zambia and in Swaziland leaves are blanched before drying (Vorster *et al.*, 2007b, p.7; Nguni & Mwila, 2007, p. 15; Masarirambi *et al.*, 2010, p.3336). Masarirambi *et al.* (2010, p.3336) goes on to explain that in Swaziland traditional vegetables are rolled into thin sheets and cut into small pieces before blanching. Blanching is extremely important in food preservation as it reduces nutrient loss, removes substances (oxalates) that are harmful to children and prevent enzymatic reaction (Masarirambi et al., 2010, p.3336; Dweba & Mearns, 2011, p.6). Furthermore in other areas, traditional vegetables are used to cook a relish, which is eaten as a side dish in addition to the staple food (Masarirambi et al., 2010, p.3337; Nesamvuni, 2000, p.89, Nguni & Mwila, 2007, p.12). Dried traditional vegetables are first soaked in water before cooking and ingredients such as garlic, onion, tomatoes, peanut butter and green pepper are added to improve flavour and nutrients that are lost during the drying process (Masarirambi et al., 2010, p.3337). However in this study dried vegetables are only used to cook porridge, a dish that was found to be less popular amongst youth and men. This means therefore that although drying of traditional vegetables might improve accessibility to traditional vegetables during dry season, some members of the community might not benefit from them and acceptable levels could be low (Dweba & Mearns, 2011, p.6). This could have negative consequences on food security because in order for food to be utilized, it should be socially acceptable to the people (McDonald, 2010, p.15).

As previously mentioned in paragraph 3 younger women were included as part of the study population to determine the potential future use of traditional vegetables. Their knowledge of traditional vegetables was used to draw conclusions about the future use of traditional vegetables. The study revealed that younger women had very little knowledge on traditional vegetables when compared to elderly women of the same village. Younger women were only able to identify 5 traditional traditional vegetables vegetables as opposed to older women who identified 33 traditional vegetables. Several researchers such as Odhav *et al.* (2007, p.430); Modi *et al.* (2006, p. 9); Lephole (2004, p. 80) and Vorster *et al.* (2007a, p. 6) arrived at a similar conclusion, noting that traditional vegetable knowledge is disappearing especially amongst youth. Furthermore, youth consumed only two traditional vegetables. Several negative statements which indicated negative attitudes surfaced during focus group discussion and these negative statements are described wholly in an article by Mearns & Dweba (2011, pp.6-7). The decline in utilization and knowledge of traditional vegetables amongst youth has been attributed to the current cooking methods used and change in taste preferences (Jansen van Rensburg, *et al.*, 2007, p. 8). Mearns & Dweba (2011, p.7) goes on to suggest other possible reasons for this decline in knowledge and consumption as being poor status associated with traditional vegetables, changes in lifestyle, education as well as urbanisation.

5. Recommendations

There were sufficient traditional vegetables available at eMantlaneni village; however they were not fully exploited to make a significant contribution towards household food security.

Traditional vegetables were accessible to respondents as the majority of them could be harvested from both cultivated landsand natural fields. Although traditional vegetables were available throughout the year in eMantlaneni village, their availability was reduced during winter and spring prior to seasonal rainfall. This would make households more vulnerable to food insecurity, due to the lower availability of traditional vegetables.

Given the evidence gathered in this study regarding the reduced consumption of traditional vegetables, it is recommended that awareness programmes about the importance of eating green leafy vegetables, therefore freely available traditional vegetables, be initiated. Awareness programmes in the form of awareness days and awareness activities that were used by Vorster et al. (2007b:7), in their study to re-create awareness of traditional leafy vegetables among communities are good examples of intervention strategies that can be initiated at eMantlaneni village to increase knowledge, status and utilization. The awareness programmes used by Vorster et al. (2007b:7) included cooking competitions, development of positive messages about traditional vegetables, plays and development of slogans, and logos that were included into all the activities. T-shirts bearing the slogans were also produced and handed over to influential people in the community. Extension workers and school learners were also involved in such awareness campaigns.

Data suggest that knowledge on post harvest activities such as cooking and preservation is limited. Therefore in order for traditional vegetables to make a significant contribution towards malnutrition and food security more attention needs to be given on developing appropriate cooking and preservation techniques that will ensure that maximum value of nutrients is elicited. These appropriate cooking and preservation techniques can then be imparted back to the community.

CONCLUSION

The research recommendations suggested that the availability and utilisation of traditional vegetables towards contributing positively to food diversity and food security are only beneficial as long as the indigenous knowledge associated with the traditional vegetables is available. The research has shown furthermore that attitudes towards the use of traditional vegetables influence the potential transfer of associated indigenous knowledge to future generations.

A multi-prolonged intervention is required if traditional vegetables are intended to be used to improve food security for resource poor rural communities. In order to motivate the use of traditional vegetables for greater food diversity further research is required to confirm the nutritional value derived from traditional vegetables. Further research on a number of cases could also be beneficial to test regional variations in utilisation of traditional vegetables and acceptable levels for traditional vegetable use.

If resource poor communities can utilise traditional vegetables as a valuable food source they have to adapt their view and attitudes towards the stigma associated with traditional vegetables and ensure the survival, sharing of, thus the conversation of indigenous knowledge associated with traditional vegetable use.

REFERENCES

Alemu, Z. G. (2010). *Measuring poverty, deprivation, and progress in service delivery: Application to the Eastern Cape Province, SA. Seminar National Agricultural Marketing Council,Pretoria*. Development Bank of Southern Africa.

Aju, P. C. & Poopola, L. (2010). The dietary role of traditional vegetables in the rural communities of Imo State, Nigeria. *Journal of Sustainable Development in Africa,* 12 (7), 104 -113

Aphane, J., Chadha, M.L. & Oluoch M.O. (2003). Increasing consumption of micronutrient-rich foods through production and promotion of indigenous foods. *In FAO- AVRDC International Workshop Proceedings*, 5-8 May 2002, Arusha, Tanzania. AVRDC- THE World Vegetable Center. Taiwan. AVRDC.

Babbie, E. (2008). *The basics of social research.* 4th ed., Belmont: Thomson Wadsworth.

Bhat, R.B. & Rhubuluza, T. (2002). The bio-diversity of traditional vegetables of the Transkei region in the Eastern Cape of South Africa. *South African Journal of Botany,* 68, 94-99.

Den Hartog, A. P., Van Staveren, W. J. & Brouwer, I.D. (2006). *Food habits and consumption in developing countries: manual for field studies.* Wageningen: Wageningen Academic Publishers.

Department of Agriculture. (2002). *Integrated food security strategy for South Africa.* Pretoria: Government Printers.

Dweba T. P. & Mearns, M. A. (2011). Conserving indigenous knowledge as the key to the current and future use of traditional vegetables. *International Journal of Information Management* (2011), doi: 10. 1016/j.ijnfomgt.2011.02.009

Eastern Cape Provincial Government (2003) *Provincial growth and development plan 2004-2014*. Policy document. Bisho. Provincial Government of the Eastern Cape.pp.18-57.

Faber, M., Laurie, S. & Venter, S. (2006) *Home-gardens to address vitamin A deficiency in South Africa: A food-based approach.* ARC Roodeplaat Vegetable and Ornamental Plant Institute,Pretoria, South Africa.

Fish, L. (1999). *Preparing herbarium specimens*. Pretoria: National Botanical Institute.

Flyman, M.V. & Afolayan, A.J. (2006). The suitability of wild vegetables for alleviating human dietary deficiencies. *South Africa Journal of Botany,* 72, 492-497.

Ingquza Hill Municipality (2007) *Integrated Development Plan 2007 /2012.*

Jansen van Rensburg, W., Van Averbeke, W., Slabbert, R., Faber, M., Van Jaarsveld, P., Van Heerden, I., Wenhold, F. & Oelofse, A. (2007a). African leafy vegetables in South Africa. *Water SA,* 33 (3), 317-326.

Jansen van Rensburg, W., Vorster, I.H.J., Van Zijl, J.J.B. & Venter, L.S. (2007b). Conservation of African leafy vegetables in South Africa. *African Journal of Food, Agriculture, Nutrition and Development*, 7(4), 1-13.

Keller, G.B., Mndiga, H. & Maass, B. L. (2005). Diversity and genetic erosion of traditional vegetables in Tanzania from the farmer's point of view. *Plant Genetic Resources,* 3(3), 400-413.

Kittler P.G. & Sucher K.P. (2000). *Cultural foods: traditions and trends*. Atlanta. Wadsworth.

Laker, M. C. (2007). African leafy vegetables in South Africa. *Water SA,* 33(3), 311-315.

Lephole, M. M. (2004). *Uses and nutritional value of traditional vegetables consumed as traditional foods in Lesotho.* Unpublished research thesis, University of the Free State, Bloemfontein, South Africa.

Masarirambi, M. T., Mavuso, V., Songwe, V. D., Nkambule, T. P. & Mhazo, N. (2010). Indigenous post-harvest handling and processing of traditional vegetables in Swaziland: A Review. *African Journal of Agricultural Research, 5 (24),* pp. 3333-3341.

McDonald B. L. (2010). *Food Security.*Cambridge. Polity Press.

Modi, M., Modi A.T. & Hendricks S. (2006). Potential role of wild vegetables in household food security: A preliminary case study in KwaZulu-Natal, South Africa. *African Journal of Food, Agriculture, Nutrition and Development,* 6(2), 1-13.

Musinguzi, E., Kikafunda, J. K. & Kiremire, B. T. (2006). Utilization of indigenous food plants in Uganda: a case study of South Western Uganda. *African Journal of Food, Agriculture, Nutrition and Development,* 6(2), 1-14.

Nesamvuni, C. (2000). *The use and nutritional value of common edible indigenous green leafy vegetables in the diet of the VhaVenda.* Unpublished master's thesis, University of the North, Polokwane, South Africa.

Nguni, D. & Mwila, G. (2007). Opportunities for increased production, utilization and income generation from African leafy vegetables in Zambia. *African Journal of Food, Agriculture, Nutrition and Development,* 7 (4), 1-20.

Odhav, B., Beekrum, S., Akula, US. & Baijnath, H. (2007). Preliminary assessment of nutritional value of traditional in KwaZulu-Natal, South Africa. *Journal of Food Composition and Analysis,* 20 (5), 430-435.

Rodriguez-Amaya, D. B., (2000) Effects of processing and storage on food carotenoids. *Sightand Life Newsletter:* Incorporating Xerophthalamia Club Bulletin. Special Issue: Many Ways,one goal, 3, pp.25-35

Rose, E. F. (1973) Some observations on the diet and farming practices of the people of the Transkei. *South African Medical Journal,*47,pp.301-303.

Shava, S. (2000). *The use of indigenous plants as food by rural community in the Eastern Cape: An educational exploration.* Unpublished master's thesis, Rhodes University, Grahamstown, South Africa.

Uusiku, N. P., Oelofse, A., Duodu, K. G., Bester, M. J. & Faber, M. (In press) (2010). Nutritional value of leafy vegetables of sub-Saharan Africa and their potential contribution to human health: A review. *Journal of Food Composition and Analysis.*

Van de Heever, E. (1995). The use and conservation of indigenous leafy vegetables. *Roodeplaat Bulletin*, 45, 16-17.

Van Vuuren, L. (2006). Wild vegetables: tamed to decrease hunger: Emerging Agriculture. *The Water Wheel*, 5, 22-25.

Viljoen, A. T., Botha, P. & Boonzaaier, C.C. (2005). Factors contributing to changes in food practices of a black South African community. *Journal of Family Ecology and Consumer Sciences*, 33, 46-62.

Vorster, I.H.J., Jansen van Rensburg, W., Van Zijl, J.J.B. & Venter, L.S. (2007a). Re-creating awareness of traditional leafy vegetables in communities. *African Journal of Food, Agriculture, Nutrition and Development*, 7(4), 1-10.

Vorster, I.H.J., Jansen van Rensburg, W., Van Zijl, J.J.B. & Venter, L.S. (2007b). The importance of traditional leafy vegetables in South Africa. *African Journal of Food, Agriculture, Nutrition and Development*, 7(4),1-13.

In: Vegetable Consumption and Health: New Research
Editors: Claudia Wilson and Melinda Morree
ISBN: 978-1-62100-941-2

Chapter 6

THE UNCANNING POWER OF EMOTIONAL BONDS: EXPLORING THE ROLE OF NOSTALGIC FOODS IN LATINAS' EATING BEHAVIORS AND HEALTH

Anahí Viladrich[1,*] and Ming-Chin Yeh[2,†]

[1]Department of Sociology, Queens College & the Graduate Center, The City University of New York, Address: 65-30 Kissena Blvd., Flushing, NY, U. S.

[2]Nutrition and Food Science Program, CUNY School of Public Health at Hunter College, Hunter College of the City University of New York, 2180 Third Av., New York, NY, U. S.

ABSTRACT

The literature has only recently begun to notice the cultural and emotional significance of familiar foods in supporting immigrants' healthy and deleterious eating practices in both their countries of origin and of destiny. The term *nostalgic foods* is used here to refer to the traditional food items and recipes prepared, eaten and maintained by immigrants and their families in the U.S., via everyday consumption and generational retention. While some aspects of traditional immigrants' diets may be protective against obesity and disease, particularly regarding the consumption of fruits and vegetables and the use of whole grains, some traditional eating patterns may be harmful, such as an excess of fried foods including chicken and plantains.

This paper underscores the results of two focus group studies conducted with Latinas in New York City (NYC). The findings revealed that participants who experienced several hurdles in a new environment, tended to feel more "at home" via the preparation and consumption of culturally familiar foods. For many of them, traditional foods from their countries of origin (either raw items as mangoes or cooked items as plantains) provided "comfort," not just because of their taste and accessibility, but because they drew powerful emotional memories of the times spent either at their countries of origin or at family gatherings in the U.S. The study underscored paradoxical results regarding the selection of both healthy items (e.g., fruits and vegetables) and unhealthy items, such as

* E-mail: anahi.viladrich@qc.cuny.edu; Phone #:718-997-2800.
† E-mail: myeh@hunter.cuny.edu; Phone #: 212-396-7776.

staples heavily loaded with sugar (*buñuelos*, a kind of fried pastries) and fat (fried chicken). Our findings underscored interesting differences between first-generation immigrants (40 years and older) and younger second-generation Latinas (between 18 and 39 years old), regarding the meanings of "authentic" foods in their lives. While the first group preferred dishes that included the same ingredients and forms of preparation utilized in their countries of origin, second generation participants concocted their own notion of the "authentic," by introducing ingredients inspired by a wide sample of ethnic foods in NYC. We conclude this chapter by proposing a few possible health intervention strategies to be considered for promoting healthy eating among immigrant and minority groups. A better understanding of Latina's preferences, preparation and utilization of nostalgic foods will likely help inform future public health interventions towards improving, and preserving, Latinas' healthy eating habits and health.

INTRODUCTION

The prevalence of obesity has reached an epidemic proportion in the U.S. According to recent statistics, approximately one-third of the U.S. adults are obese. Ethnic minority populations, such as Hispanics (or Latinos) [1], are most severely affected by this debilitating condition. They also experience higher rates of obesity than their white counterparts (Flegal, Carroll, Ogden, and Curtin, 2010). Obesity varies according to age as well. For instance, in a study conducted on women 60 years and older, it was found that 37% of Mexican-American women were obese compared with 32% of non-Hispanic White women, but approximately 51% of Mexican-American women 40–59 years of age were obese compared with about 39% of non-Hispanic White women of the same age (Ogden, Carroll, McDowell, Flegal, 2007).

The literature also reports that first-generation Latinas tend to weigh less and have a better health status than do their non-Latina White counterparts; although long-term first-generation Latinas and those of subsequent generations present a higher prevalence of obesity (Popkin and Udry, 1998).

Focusing on the health of Hispanics in the US is crucial to our understanding of the morbidity and mortality trends of the country at large. Not only are Hispanics the largest minority group in the US, but their proportion is expected to double by the year 2050, when they will become nearly 25% of the population (Henry J. Kaiser Family Foundation, 2003). In New York City (NYC), Latinos comprise 27% of the US population —the second largest group after non-Hispanic Whites (35% of the population, Fund for Public Health in New York, 2004). Furthermore, Latinos present significantly high rates of obesity and weight-related issues, including diabetes and cardiovascular disease in the US. (Yeh, Viladrich, Roy, Bruning, 2009). As a result, obesity among this population has become the tip of the iceberg that reveals the growing pervasive impact of chronic conditions among minority groups, which are linked to social and racial inequalities (Viladrich, 2009).

Rising obesity trends are also strikingly associated with the increasing consumption of high-calorie, low-nutrient foods in place of healthier staples, which in many cases are out of the reach of the urban poor. In this vein, there has been an increasing interest in understanding the role of cultural habits in shaping both healthy and deleterious nutritional patterns among diverse ethnic populations in the U.S., including Hispanic sub-groups (Viladrich, 2009).

---

[1] In this chapter, we use the terms Hispanics and Latinos interchangeably.

The literature has only recently begun to notice the cultural and emotional significance of familiar foods in supporting immigrants' harmful eating practices, which may contribute to the growing trends in obesity among specific minority populations in the U.S. (Koc and Welsh, 2001; Locher, Yoels, Maurer, van Ells., 2005).

The examination of Latinas' eating preferences and nutritional patterns may be key to the designing and development of successful health promotion interventions, including weight-control and healthy eating programs, addressed to this population. In order to examine Latinas' nutritional beliefs and food choices in the U.S., this chapter first discusses the significant health effects of fruit and vegetable consumption. We then introduce the concept of "nostalgic foods" by examining the evidence drawn from our recent focus group studies conducted with Latina immigrants (Viladrich, Yeh, Bruning, Weiss, 2009; Viladrich, 2009; Tagliaferro, Herman, Bruning, Wong, Nguyen, Saini and Viladrich, 2010).

The results from these studies provide striking evidence on the importance of culturally familiar foods in shaping Latinas' food preferences and their eating patterns in the US.[2] Finally, we conclude by providing several strategies for promoting fruit and vegetable consumption among Latinos and other minority groups in the US, which have meaningful policy implications for the health of the U.S. population in general and of Latino groups in particular.

Fruits and Vegetables as Nostalgic Memorabilia

Fruits and vegetables consumption is found to be protective against cardiovascular disease, type 2 diabetes, metabolic syndrome, and certain types of cancer (Steinmetz and Potter, 1996; Feldeisen and Tucker, 2007; Ford and Mokdad, 2001). In addition, consumption of fruits and vegetables is associated with a decreased risk for obesity and improved weight management (He, Hu, Colditz, Manson, Willett, Liu, 2004; Bazzano, 2006). A recent study involving three separate cohorts that included 120,877 U.S. women and men has found that increased daily servings of fruits and vegetables was indeed associated with weight loss (Mozaffarian, Hao, Rimm, Willett, Hu, 2011). A healthy diet generally includes an abundant amount of fruits and vegetables. However, the majority of Americans do not eat the amounts recommended as part of healthy dietary patterns (CDC, 2007).

While Hispanics have reported higher intakes of fruits and vegetables than Whites and African-Americans (Thompson, Midthune, Subar, McNeel, Berrigan, Kipnis, 2005), it has also been shown that those more acculturated (usually long-term immigrants and second generation individuals) tend to consume lower amounts than recent immigrants (Gregory-Mercado, Staten, Ranger-Moore, Thomson, Will, Ford, et al, 2006). Although these results suggest the important role acculturation plays in immigrants' diet, more information is needed in order to understand sub-groups' differences regarding food preferences and their changes in eating behaviors upon arrival in the host societies (Yeh, et al., 2009). With rates of obesity

[2] Two focus-group studies were conducted with first- and second-generation Hispanic women in the years 2006-07 and 2010. The first one (led by Dr. Viladrich and Dr. Yeh) was sponsored by the George N. Shuster Faculty Fellowship Fund at Hunter College. The second study (conducted by Dr. Viladrich) was awarded a grant by the Professional Staff Congress Grant (PSC) CUNY. Both research projects shared the common goal of examining women's food preferences and their belief towards the consumption of healthy foods, their overall nutrition patterns and their perceived barriers to physical activity in the US.

and chronic diseases on the rise especially among minority and immigrant populations, the nostalgic concept of food warrants further exploration.

Many immigrants carry the images of their favorite recipes from their home countries. Latino immigrants, who often experience several hurdles in a new environment, tend to feel more "at home" via the preparation and consumption of culturally familiar foods (Tagliaferro, et al, 2010; Viladrich, 2009). It is possible that these food memories play a crucial role in keeping (and adopting) certain eating patterns with their consequent health effects, either protective or harmful, after immigrants' arrival in the societies of reception. The nostalgic feeling associated with certain food items could explain, in part, immigrants' maintenance of specific eating practices after their arrival in the U.S. Fruits and vegetables, in this instance, could serve as part of the "nostalgic memorabilia" that brings immigrants closer to their countries of birth while residing in the host society. Nevertheless, other traditional dietary practices may not be conducive to healthy eating. In the following section, we provide some context for the definition and utilization of the "nostalgic foods" concept framed by the results of two focus group studies conducted with Hispanic women in NYC.

The Meanings of Nostalgia

The term "nostalgic foods" is used here to refer to the traditional food items and recipes prepared, eaten and maintained by immigrants and their families in the U.S., via everyday consumption and generational retention. Despite the fact that a large literature exists on the emotional bonding that links immigrants to the foods from their countries of origin, there is still scarce evidence on how these are consumed, and transformed, in recipient societies, as well as on their impact on immigrants' health (Viladrich, 2009). A main aspect involved with the preference for, and choice of, nostalgic foods relates to the collective construction of ethnic identity, as a powerful community bond regardless of Latinos' countries of origin. Immigrants' longing for particular staples is ingrained in their need for cultural and familial protection that may be useful to alleviate feelings of homesickness, vulnerability and high levels of stress that are often experienced in the host environment (Locher et al., 2005). Latino immigrants, who often experience several hurdles in a new environment, tend to recreate their cultures of origin via the preparation and consumption of culturally familiar foods (Koc and Welsh, 2001). We argue that while some aspects of traditional immigrants' diets may be protective against obesity and chronic diseases, particularly regarding the use of whole grains and legumes often included in the preparation of corn bread, tortillas, beans, and rice (Dixon, Sundquist, Winkleby, 2000); some traditional eating patterns may be harmful, including an excess of fried foods such as chicken and plantains (Brand-Miller, Holt, Pawlak, McMillan, 2002).

Our research findings based on a focus group methodology (Viladrich, et al., 2009; Viladrich, 2009; Tagliaferro, et al., 2010) provided a deeper understanding of Latinas' eating habits in relation to their food preferences, nutritional choices and weight management, including their reliance on specific nostalgic foods. For most study participants, traditional foods from their countries of origin (either raw items as mangoes or cooked items like *plantains*) provided "comfort," not just because of their taste and accessibility, but because they drew powerful emotional memories of the times spent either at their countries of origin or at family gatherings in the U.S.

Latina participants reported having access to fruits such as mangos and watermelons in their backyards back home. They also mentioned that they could easily buy them anywhere on the street. Therefore, by preparing, eating and sharing familiar foods, women were able to recreate strong emotional connections with those they loved both in the U.S. and in their countries of birth. Nevertheless, due to high costs, inaccessibility and other barriers, many of our participants were not able to consume healthy foods in the U.S. regularly. Instead, they reported a tendency to replace them with processed and sugary foods (e.g., pastries) that are cheap, ready to eat and perceived to be tasty overall (Viladrich, David, Yeh, Bruning, 2008). This negative aspect of food nostalgia could prove detrimental to their health.

BETWEEN COMMON EXPERIENCES AND INNER DIFFERENCES

Latinas' emotional attachment to nostalgic foods, as a means to keep the image of their native countries alive, is a multi-fold concept that varies according to their countries of origin, generation and age. Our study results underscore interesting differences between first-generation immigrants (40 years and older) and younger second-generation Latinas (between 18 and 39 years old), regarding the meanings of nostalgic foods in their lives. First-generation Latinas seem to be more likely to consume traditional diverse diets, a fact that may partially explain their initial healthier weight and health status, which deteriorates over time (Aldrich and Variyam, 2000; Viladrich, et al., 2008).

A related matter is linked to the genuine origin and authenticity of the produces and spices utilized, for which women expressed different stances in our studies. First generation Latinas drew powerful images regarding the emotional memory of what (and how) they used to eat in their countries of origin. These representations became a powerful reminder of the importance of keeping their traditional foods alive—as they were prepared and ate at home. Older women aimed at conserving their dishes' original recipes as much as possible by using the same ingredients, their familiar seasonings and the forms of preparation they learned and utilized in their countries of birth. During the focus groups, we were surprised to hear that some study participants would bring (or import) some food staples that are actually easily found in the U.S.—at cheaper prices in some cases. Some women proudly narrated the unusual efforts they would make to carry raw staples (e.g., beans or shrimp) or cooked items (e.g., *tortillas*) from their countries of origin.

Furthermore, older women tended to cook traditional foods daily (not just during special celebrations), and therefore had a prominent role in shaping the culinary *habitus* of their families (Bourdieu, 1984), which was expressed in their eagerness to keep alive the tastes and flavors of the typical foods that they consumed in their countries of origin. The overall conclusion from the above studies is that first-generation Latinas often function as "food gatekeepers," culture transmitters, and role models for other members of their families, especially their daughters (Yeh, et al., 2009). Additionally, for older first generation Latinas (mothers, grandmothers, aunts), feeding others may be a primary way of showing their love and care for family members, as well as a means of passing beliefs and values of their culture of origin to the next generation.

Second generation Latinas in our studies, however, revealed a more complex relationship to nostalgic foods. While on the one hand they tended to incorporate multi-ethnic choices to their food preferences; on the other, they were more innovative when it came to experimenting with new ingredients and forms of preparation, as in the case of finding substitutes (such as using olive oil instead of fat, and baking instead of frying) in order to make their food preparations healthier. Fusion cuisine and ethnic innovation were two of the characteristics that represented younger women's food choices, which did not necessarily homologize the recipes found in their countries of origin. These younger participants seemed more open to the idea of experimenting between cultures; therefore they were not hooked on reproducing the home cooking they grew up with, but were eager to incorporating novel culinary trends that they would find in the multi-cultural urban milieu.

BUILDING A COMMON GROUND

Regardless of age and recency in the U.S., all participants expressed a nostalgic attachment to tropical fruits as an *organic cornucopia*, which was translated into representations of cleaned and natural environments where everybody has access to fruits and vegetables that may be gathered in one's "own backyard" (Tagliaferro, et al., 2010). In addition, most women shared a deep concern about chemically processed foods in the U.S., and their belief that it is easier (and cheaper) to find and buy natural and healthy foods back home. Furthermore, Latina participants seemed to agree with that the underlying reason for much of their weight gain in the U.S. is intrinsically related to the ways in which most foods (e.g., fruits, vegetables and meats) are grown and processed in this country. The typical example they provided was illustrated by "the hormone-injected poultry" image, which has an alleged effect on Latinas' increasing obesity trends in the U.S. On the contrary, most women reported that fruits and vegetables are pesticide- and hormone-free back home, and therefore lack the weight-gaining effect that characterize them in the U.S.

Additionally, both first- and second-generation participants identified common obstacles in their access to fruits and vegetables, which are rooted in their higher prices and inaccessibility in the urban milieu. As a result, much of Latinas' retained eating habits seemed to be biased against healthy staples and towards less healthy ones. Our results suggest that, for the most part, study participants were clearly aware of the structural factors that prevented them from "eating well" in the U.S. For instance, respondents mentioned the high stress levels they experienced daily —typically framed as the direct effect of their hectic job schedules and their multiple family obligations, which led them to craving for sugar-loaded sweets (e.g., cookies, doughnuts and muffins). These food items are not only cheaper than vegetables and fruits, but are also easier to find and buy everywhere in NYC. Some women even complained about the changes in the urban environment, which in NYC has been boosted by gentrification forces. As a result, the "food desert" (in the form of scarcity of healthy food choices often experienced in inner cities) characterizes much of the study participants' concerns about the shifting geography of the built environment in their neighborhoods. The higher prices of fruits and vegetables in many NYC's neighborhoods have created stronger barriers to Latinas' consumption of fruits and vegetables vis-à-vis their easy access to ubiquitous junk foods.

Finally, most women mentioned changes in their life styles in the U.S., expressed in the tendency to work long hours and take public transportation, instead of walking, amid the little time they routinely have for the preparation of vegetables and grains— a trend that typically led them to rely on processed foods (e.g., pizza) which are mouth-watering and easy to buy. As a result, even among study participants who were quite aware of the importance of consuming fruits and vegetables, they tended to report eating patterns that favored energy-dense, high-caloric foods (e.g., fried chicken or chips). In the end, participants' romanticization of the nostalgic and natural foods they had at home represented a *resilient effect* aimed at reckoning their discomfort with the barriers to healthy eating they experienced in the U.S.

CONCLUSION

This chapter has introduced the concept of nostalgic foods for the purpose of defining the traditional food items and recipes prepared, eaten and maintained by Latina immigrants and their families in the U.S., via everyday consumption and generational retention. Our results bring a contribution in the direction of underscoring the importance of the emotional significance of familiar foods in immigrants' healthy eating practices in the U.S. As noted earlier, while some aspects of traditional immigrants' diets may be protective against obesity and chronic diseases, some other nostalgic patterns may be harmful, such as an excess intake of fried items and processed foods. The examination of the meaning and utilization of nostalgic foods among Latinas underscores paradoxical results regarding the selection of both healthy items (e.g., fruits and vegetables) and unhealthy ones, including foods that are heavily loaded with sugar (*buñuelos*, a kind of fried pastries) and fat (fried chicken).

Another relevant finding in this study evokes the notion of "authenticity," that is expressed in Latinas' choice of food staples considered to be genuine expressions of their cultures of origin. This notion seems to play a key role in shaping Latina immigrants' food preferences that also diverges along generational lines. On the one hand, first generation Latina participants reported seeking nostalgic foods in their local ethnic neighborhoods, or to the extent possible, bring those foods from their countries of origin. On the other hand, second generation participants tended to concoct their own notion of the authentic recipes inspired by a wide sample of ethnic foods in NYC. A better understanding of Latinas' food preferences, amid the preparation and consumption of nostalgic foods, will likely help inform future public health interventions towards improving, and preserving, Latinas' healthy eating habits in the U.S.

Despite of the qualitative nature of this study, which does not attempt to be generalizable to the larger Latino populations in NYC or in the U.S., our results coincide with those of a similar study (based on a mixed quantitative-qualitative methodology) conducted by Park and colleagues (2011) on Hispanic women's dietary practices.[3] Park and colleagues concluded that their participants' concerns about freshness and purity, represented by the absence of chemicals and preservatives, were the primary categories they used to define healthy foods. In

[3] When conducting focus group studies, a careful interpretation of the results is recommended regarding the differences between what participants express as their ideal behaviors and what they actual practices are, particularly when it comes to their food choices and actual eating trends (Betts, 2006).

agreement with our findings, the authors concluded that the existence of fresh products (e.g., from local farms) could have a beneficial effect on the nutritional patterns of Latinas living in the urban milieu.

Undoubtedly, much remains to be learned about the role of nostalgic foods in Latinas' day-to-day eating practices, the cultural beliefs out of which they arise, and the potential impact of culinary traditions on Latino families' health. Although recent interventions have taken into consideration the relevance and persistence of immigrants' customary eating practices, a deeper and broader understanding of the role of nostalgic foods will help inform public health interventions aiming at slowing, and reversing, the rising trends in obesity and related diseases among immigrants in the U.S. (Gordon-Larsen, et al. 2003, Palmieri, et al., 1998).

To end this chapter, we propose several health intervention strategies to be considered for promoting healthy eating among immigrant and minority groups. They include: 1) making fruits and vegetables more available and accessible to Hispanics and their families by subsidizing the price of fruits and vegetables through bodegas, neighborhood markets and local farms that sell them; 2) providing healthy recipes written in Spanish that rely on seasonal and locally grown produces. In this vein, some of our interviewees proposed meaningful and easy ways to improving Latinos' eating practices. Small changes to food preparation such as baking instead of frying, and choosing low-fat versions of many processed foods are deemed feasible and practical; 3) supporting promotional campaigns sponsored by local community organizations or health departments emphasizing the advantages of eating fruits and vegetables; 4) taking advantage of immigrants' natural sites where they gather on a routine basis. For instance, bodegas, beauty parlors and churches can offer unique opportunities for health promotion programs and disease prevention interventions. As such, relying on lay advisors and *promotoras de salud* (health lay advisors) can provide a meaningful vehicle for disseminating food alternatives among Latina women in the U.S. Finally, community programs (rather than individual-centered interventions) will be more effective in improving the nutritional patterns of disenfranchised immigrant populations, including Latinas in the U.S.

Acknowledgements

The authors wish to acknowledge the participation of Nancy Bruning (research associate and project coordinator) and of the following research assistants in the data-collection process and initial analysis of the study results (in alphabetical order): Stephanie Herman, Linda Nguyen, Isha Saini, Barbara Tagliaferro and Kim Wong. This study was supported in part by PSC-CUNY grants, # 68770-00 37 and # 68747-00 37 and by a George N. Shuster Faculty Fellowship Fund.

REFERENCES

Aldrich, L., Variyam, J. N. (2000). Acculturation erodes the diet quality of U.S. Hispanics. *Food Review*, 23(1): 51-55.

Bazzano L. (2006). The high cost of not consuming fruits and vegetables. *Journal of the American Dietetic Association*, 106:1364-1368.

Betts, N., T. Baranowski, et al. (1996). Recommendations for planning and reporting focus group research. *Journal of Nutrition Education and Behavior,* 28: 279-81.

Brand-Miller, J., Holt, S., Pawlak, D.B., McMillan, J. (2002). Glycemic index and obesity. *The American Journal of Clinical Nutrition,* 76(suppl): 281S-285S.

Bourdieu, P. (1984). *Distinction : A social critique of the judgement of taste.* Cambridge: Harvard University Press.

Centers for Disease Control and Prevention. (2007). Fruit and vegetable consumption among adults—United States, 2005. *Morbidity and Mortality Weekly Report;* 56, 213-217.

Dixon, L. B., Sundquist, J., Winkleby, M. (2000). Differences in energy, nutrient, and food intakes in a US sample of Mexican-American women and men: findings from the Third National Health and Nutrition Examination Survey, 1988-1994. *American Journal of Epidemiology* 152(6): 548-557.

Feldeisen, S. E., Tucker, K.L. (2007). Nutritional strategies in the prevention and treatment of metabolic syndrome. *Applied Physiology, Nutrition and Metabolism,* 32:46-60.

Flegal, K. M., Carroll, M. D., Ogden, C. L., and Curtin, L. R. (2010). Prevalence and trends in obesity among US adults, 1999-2008. *Journal of the American Medical Association,* 303(3), 235e241.

Ford ES, Mokdad AH. (2001). Fruit and vegetable consumption and diabetes mellitus incidence among US adults. *Preventive Medicine,* 32:33-39.

Fund for Public Health in New York. (2004). Health disparities in New York City. Available at: http://www.nyc.gov/html/doh/pdf/epi/disparities-2004.pdf.

Gordon-Larsen, P., K. M. Harris, et al. (2003). Acculturation and overweight-related behaviors among Hispanic immigrants to the US: the National Longitudinal Study of Adolescent Health. *Social Science and Medicine* 57(11):2023-34.

Gregory-Mercado, K.Y., Staten, L.K., Ranger-Moore, J., Thomson, C.A., Will, J.C., Ford, E.S., Guillen, J., Larkey, L.K, Giuliano, A.R., and Marshall, J. (2006). Fruit and vegetable consumption of older Mexican-American women is associated with their acculturation level. *Ethnicity and Disease,* 16,89-95.

He, K., Hu, F.B., Colditz, G.A., Manson, J.E., Willett, W.C., Liu, S. (2004). Changes in intake of fruits and vegetables in relation to risk of obesity and weight gain among middle-aged women. *International Journal of Obesity Related Metabollic Disorder,* ;28:1569-1574.

Henry J Kaiser Family Foundation. (2003). Key facts: race, ethnicity, and medical care, from http://www.kff.org/minorityhealth/upload/Key-Facts-Race-Ethnicity-Medical-Care-Chartbook.pdf.

Koc, M. and J. Welsh (2001). *Food, identity and the immigrant experience. Ethnocultural, racial, religious, and linguistic diversity and identity seminar*. Halifax, Nova Scotia.

Locher, J. L.,Yoels, W.C., Maurer, D., van Ells, J. (2005). Comfort foods: an exploratory journey into the social and emotional significance of food. *Food and Foodways*, (13): 273-297.

Mozaffarian, D., Hao, T., Rimm, E.B., Willett, W.C., Hu, F.B. (2011). Changes in diet and lifestyle and long-term weight gain in women and men. *New England Journal of Medicine* 23;364(25):2392-404.

Ogden, C. L., Carroll M.D., McDowell, M.A., Flegal, K.M. (2007). Obesity among adults in the United States— no change since 2003–2004. NCHS data brief no 1. Hyattsville, MD, National Center for Health Statistics.

Palmeri, D., Auld, G. W., Taylor, T., Kendall, P., Anderson J. (1998). Multiple Perspectives on Nutrition Education Needs of Low-Income Hispanics. *Journal of Community Health* 23: 301-16.

Park, Y, Quinn J, Florez, K., Jacobson, J., Neckerman, K., Rundle, A. (2011). Hispanic immigrant women's perspective on healthy foods and the New York City retail food environment: A mixed-method study. *Social Science and Medicine* 73, 13-21.

Popkin BM., Udry, JR. (1998) Adolescent obesity increases significantly in second and third generation US Immigrants: The National Longitudinal Study of Adolescent Health, *Journal of Nutrition* 128(4):701-706.

Steinmetz KA, Potter JD. (1996). Vegetables, fruit, and cancer prevention: a review. *Journal of the American Dietetic Association,* 96:1027-1039.

Tagliaferro, B., Herman, S., Bruning, N., Wong, K., Nguyen, L., Saini I., and Viladrich, A. (2010). Nostalgic foods: the good and the bad, the raw and the cooked. *Anthropology News,* 2010, 37-38.

Thompson, F.E., Midthune D., Subar A.F., McNeel T., Berrigan D., Kipnis, V. (2005). Dietary intake estimates in the National Health Interview Survey, 2000: methodology, results and interpretation. *Journal of the American Dietetic Association,* 105, 352-363.

Viladrich, A., David D., Yeh, MC., Bruning, N. (2008). Addressing Latinas' double jeopardies: the challenge of nostalgic foods in promoting healthy eating patterns in the US. *APHA Annual Meeting*, San Diego.

Viladrich, A (2009) Maria's dilemma: between nostalgia and healthy foods. *Anthropology News*, 50(5):45-46.

Viladrich, A., Yeh, MC., Bruning, N., Weiss, R. (2009) Do real women have curves? Paradoxical body images among Latinas in New York City. *Journal of Immigrant and Minority Health*, 2009a; 11:20-28.

Yeh, MC., Viladrich, A., Roy, C., Bruning, N. (2009) Determinants of Latina obesity in the US: The role of selective acculturation. *Journal of Transcultural Nursing*, 20:105-115.

In: Vegetable Consumption and Health: New Research
Editors: Claudia Wilson and Melinda Morree
ISBN: 978-1-62100-941-2

Chapter 7

CUCUMBER AS A SOURCE OF BIOLOGICAL ACTIVE SUBSTANCES

Hisashi Kato-Noguchi and Ho Le Thi
Department of Applied Biological Science,
Faculty of Agriculture, Kagawa University, Miki, Kagawa, Japan

ABSTRACT

Cucumber (*Cucumis sativus* L.) is cultivated widely as a vegetable crop. However, major parts of plants, such as stems, leaves and roots are mostly dumped as wastes at large expense after crop harvesting. Plants produce hundreds of secondary compounds and allelopathic active substances were found in cucumber plants. Allelopathic substance can provide a competitive advantage for host-plants through suppression of soil microorganism and inhibition of the growth of competing plant species because of their antibacterial, antifungal, and growth inhibitory activities. Allelopathy may represent a new frontier for the implementation of the practices applicable in the sustainable weed management strategies. In addition, allelopathic substances have potential as either herbicides or templates for new herbicide classes because of their strong herbicidal activity.

Keywords: Allelopathy; biological active compound, cucumber waste, sustainable agriculture

INTRODUCTION

Cucumber (*Cucumis sativus* L.) is one of the important crop plants in the gourd family Cucurbitaceae and cultivated widely as a vegetable crop. The fruit is used not only food, but also in folk medicines and folk cosmetics. The stem, leaves and roots are also used in folk medicine as anti-diarrheal, detoxicant and anti-gonorrheal agents (Potter and Steinmetz, 1996; Jamir et al., 1999; Aburjai and Natsheh, 2003). Therefore, cucumber plants may contain several important biological active compounds. However, the constitutions of these compounds are not fully understood. Major parts of cucumber plants, such as stems, leaves and roots are mostly dumped as large wastes at large expense after crop harvesting. The manipulation of wastes is now becoming a serious environmental issue. It is worthwhile seeking how to make use of the waste of the cucumber.

The extracts of cucumber plant wastes inhibited the germination and growth of *Echinochloa crus-galli* under laboratory and greenhouse conditions (Thi et al., 2008a). *E. crus-galli* is one of the most significant biological constraints to agricultural crop production in many counties (Chin, 2001; Xuan et al., 2006). These findings suggest that cucumber plants may have substances with allelopathic activity. In addition, cucumber plants have been reported to secrete unknown allelochemicals from their roots into their rhizosphere (Putnam and Duke, 1974; Yu and Matsui, 1994; Yu et al., 2003).

Allelopathy is one expression of the biological phenomenon of chemical interaction and is probably of widespread significance in the functioning of natural plant communities (Seigler, 1996; Einhelling, 1999; Dayan et al., 2000). Allelochemicals are such organic chemicals involved in the allelopathy. The chemicals can provide a competitive advantage for host-plants through suppression of soil microorganism and inhibition of the growth of competing plant species because of their antibacterial, antifungal, and growth inhibitory activities (McClly, 1999; Hawes et al., 2000; Bais et al., 2006; Belz, 2007).

Allelochemicals have potential as either herbicides or templates for new herbicide classes because of their growth inhibitory activity (Duke, 1986; Putnam, 1988; Gross and Parthier, 1994; Seigler, 1996; Duke et al., 2000; Macías et al., 2007). Over many years, various types of allelochemicals have been isolated and characterized from hundreds of plant species (Rice, 1984; Dodge, 1987; Rizvi and Rizvi, 1992; Narwal, 1999). However, the information about allelochemicals in cucumber plants is limited. In this chapter, the allelopathic potential of the cucumber plants, and three allelopathic substances in the cucumber plants were described. Biological activities and endogenous levels of these substances in cucumber plants were also summarized.

Biological Activity of Cucumber Plants

Cucumber (*Cucumis sativus* L. cv. Phung Tuong) plants (including stems, leaves and roots) were obtained from the field in Cuu Long Delta, Vietnam after the final crop harvesting and dried at 50 °C for 3 days. Dry cucumber plants were soaked in the water and the biological activity of the soaked solution was determined (Table 1). The soaked solution inhibited germination, and growth of shoots, roots and fresh mass of *E. crus-galli* under Petri dish condition.

These inhibitions were increased with the increasing soaking periods of cucumber plants until 9 days and decreased thereafter. These results indicate that growth inhibiting substances may be leached and accumulated in soaking solution, but degradation of these substances may be faster than their accumulation after 9 days.

The inhibitions in respect to germination, and growth of shoots, roots and fresh mass of *E. crus-galli* were also increased with the increasing extract concentration of cucumber plants (Table 2). Significant interaction between concentrations and soaking periods was found. Higher extract concentrations gave greater inhibition at each soaking periods. The maximum inhibiting effect was found in the extract at the concentration of 5.33 g L^{-1} with 9 day-soaking.

Table 1. Effects of soaking periods of cucumber on germination and growth of barnyard grass (Thi et al., 2008a)

Soaking periods (day)	Germination (%)	Shoot length (mm)	Root length (mm)	Flesh weight (mg/Petri dish)
0	75.3 a	49.6 a	45.5 a	762 a
3	52.6 b	29.1 c	10.5 b	252 d
5	44.4 c	26.6 e	8.9 bc	297 c
7	33.9 e	22.2 f	6.5 de	217 de
9	29.4 f	20.5 g	6.3 e	199 e
11	36.5 de	23.0 f	7.1 cde	246 d
13	39.2 d	27.9 d	7.9 cde	289 c
15	39.5 d	32.3 b	7.6 cde	297 c
17	49.2 b	33.3 b	8.6 cde	346 b

Dry cucumber plants (4.0 g) were soaked in water (1 L) for 0 -17 days. After soaking, supernatant (10 mL) of these water extracts was added onto filter paper in a 10-cm Petri dish, and 100 seeds of *Echinochloa crus-galli* were sown on the filter paper. After 15 days incubation at room temperature (about 28 °C), germination percentage, plant height, root length, fresh weight of *E. crus-galli* were determined. Experiments were repeated four times in completely randomized block design. Means followed by same letters in each column are not significantly different at 5% level.

Table 2. Effects of soaking concentration of cucumber on germination and growth of *Echinochloa crus-galli* (Thi et al., 2008a)

Concentration (g/L)	Germination (%)	Shoot length (mm)	Root length (mm)	Fresh weight (mg/Petri dish)
0	78.3 a	49.7 a	47.4 a	771 a
2.67	36.4 b	22.1 b	10.9 b	218 b
4.00	29.4 c	20.5 c	6.3 c	199 c
5.33	20.9 d	17.2 d	2.5 d	132 d

Dried cucumber plants were soaked in distilled water in the ratio of 0, 2.67, 4.00 and 5.33 g dry cucumber to 1 L of distilled water for 9 days. The biological activity of the supernatant was determined as described in Table 1. Other detail as for Table 1.

Biological activity of the powder of cucumber plants was determined (Table 3). The powder significantly inhibited germination and tiller number of *E. crus-galli* under greenhouse conditions. These inhibitions were increased with the increasing application of cucumber powder, which suggests that allelopathic substances may be leached from cucumber powders into soils. The concentrations of 4.91, 9.82, 14.73, 19.64 and 24.55 g cucumber powder per pot, respectively, corresponded to 2, 3, 4, 5 and 6 tons of cucumber powder per one hectare.

Table 3. Effects of dosage of cucumber powder on germination and growth of *Echinochloa crus-galli* (Thi et al., 2008a)

Powder (g /pot)	Germination (%)	Tiller number per pot	
	Day 8	Day 14	Day 42
0	85.0 a	20.3 a	32.0 a
4.91	75.0 ab	18.4 ab	30.9 ab
9.82	67.5 bc	18.1 ab	29.6 ab
14.73	65.0 bc	17.6 bc	29.1 abc
19.64	55.0 cd	14.7 d	29.0 abc
24.55	45.0 d	11.7 e	24.9 c

Dried cucumber plants were powdered and spread over soil surface of the pots at 4.81, 9.82, 14.73, 19.64 and 24.55 g cucumber powder per pot. After watering, these pots were kept in a greenhouse for 9 days. Then, 20 seeds of *E. crus-galli* were sown in the pots. Water was supplied adequately. Germination rate of *E. crus-galli* was determined at day 8 after sowing, tillers of *E. crus-galli* were counted at day 14 and 42 after sowing. Other detail as for Table 1.

Water extract and powder of cucumber plants inhibited germination and growth of *E. crus-galli* under Petri dish and greenhouse conditions. These inhibitions were increased with the increasing soaking periods of cucumber plants in water until 9 days (Table 1), with the increasing extract concentrations of cucumber plants (Table 2), and with the increasing powder application of cucumber plants (Table 3). These results suggest that some allelopathic substances may be leached from cucumber plants into water and soils, and act as allelochemicals.

Allelopathic Activity of Cucumber Extracts

Cucumber plants were extracted with aqueous methanol and biological activity of the extract was determined by test plant species (Figure 1). The extract of cucumber plants inhibited root and shoot growth of all the species including weed species (crabgrass, *E. crus-galli* and *E. colonum*), and increasing the extract concentration increased the inhibition.

The extract obtained from 0.3 g dry weight cucumber plants inhibited the root growth of cress, lettuce, alfalfa, ryegrass, timothy, crabgrass, *E. crus-galli* and *E. colonum* by 97.7, 90.4, 95.5, 100, 100, 98.8, 96.3 and 90.7 %, respectively, and inhibited the shoot growth of cress, lettuce, alfalfa, ryegrass, timothy, crabgrass, *E. crus-galli* and *E. colonum* by 95.3, 80, 93.2, 100, 87, 88, 58 and 52 %, respectively. Thus, the aqueous methanol extract of cucumber plants may contains allelopathic substances.

Separation and Isolation of Allelopathic Substances

The aqueous methanol extract of cucumber plants was divided into ethyl acetate and aqueous fractions, and their biological activities were determined. Both fractions suppressed root and shoot growth of cress seedlings (Figure 2). However, inhibitory activity of the ethyl acetate fraction was greater than that of the aqueous fraction. Thus, the ethyl acetate fraction was further separated by a silica gel column chromatography and eluted with *n*-hexane containing increasing amounts of ethyl acetate and methanol. Inhibitory activity was found in Fractions 8 and10 (Figure 3). Fraction 8 was further purified by Sephadex LH-20, C_{18} Sep-Pak cartridges, and HPLC, and two allelopathic substances **1** and **2** were isolated as colorless oil (Thi et al., 2008b; Kato-Noguchi et al., 2011). Fraction 10 was also further purified by Sephadex LH-20, C_{18} Sep-Pak cartridges, and HPLC, and an alleloapthic substance **3** was isolated as colorless oil (Kato-Noguchi et al., 2011).

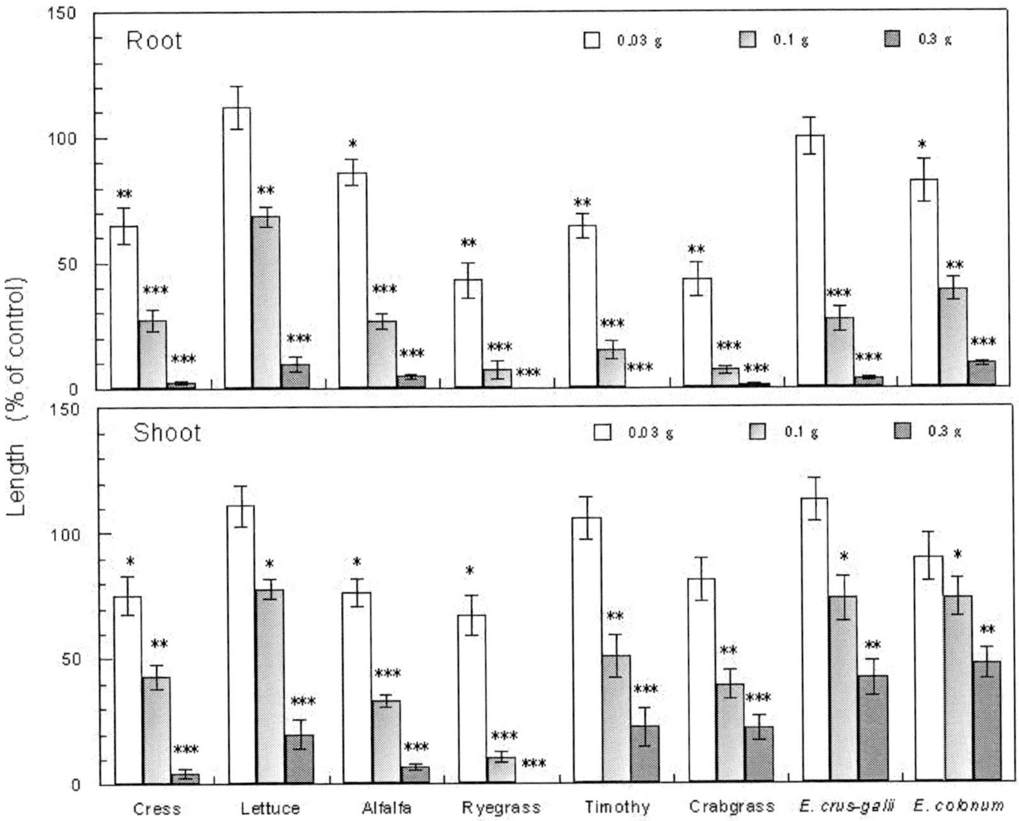

Figure 1. Effects of aqueous methanol extract of cucumber plants on root and shoot growth of cress, lettuce, alfalfa, ryegrass, timothy, crabgrass, *Echinochloa crus-galli* and *E. colonum* (Thi et al., 2008b). Dried cucumber plants were extracted with aqueous cold methanol for two days. After filtration, the extract was evaporated to dryness, dissolved in a 0.2 ml of methanol and added to a sheet of filter paper in a Petri dish. The methanol was evaporated and the filter paper in the Petri dishes was moistened with 0.05% (v/v) aqueous solution of Tween 20. After germination, 10 seeds of cress (*Lepidium sativum* L.), lettuce (*Lactuca sativa* L.), alfalfa (*Medicago sativa* L.), ryegrass (*Lolium multiflorum* L.), timothy (*Phleum pratense* L.), crabgrass (*Digitaria sanguinalis* L.), *Echinochloa crus-galli* (L.) Beauv or *Echinochloa colonum* (L.) Link were then placed into the Petri dishes. The length of their shoots and roots was measured after 48 h of incubation in the darkness at 25 °C. Concentrations of tested samples corresponded to the extract obtained from 0.03, 0.1 and 0.3 g dry weight cucumber plants. Means ± SE from 3 independent experiments with 10 plants for each determination are shown. Asterisk indicates significant difference between control and treatment: *, $P < 0.05$, **, $P < 0.01$, ***, $P < 0.001$.

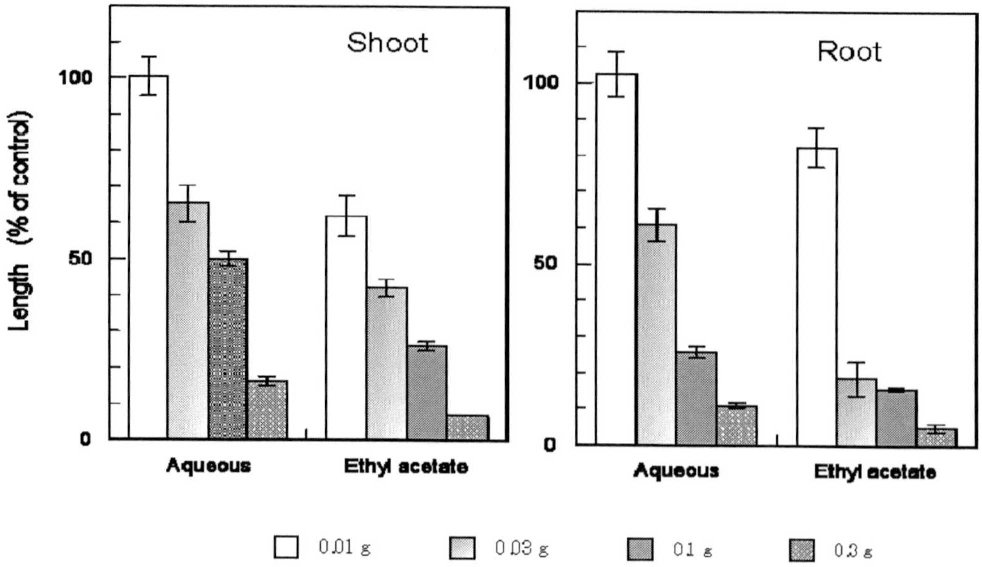

Figure 2. Effects of ethyl acetate and aqueous fraction isolated from an aqueous methanol extract of cucumber plants on root and shoot growth of cress (Thi et al., 2008b). Concentrations of tested samples corresponded to the extract obtained from 0.01, 0.03, 0.1 and 0.3 g dry weight cucumber plants. Other detail as for Figure 1.

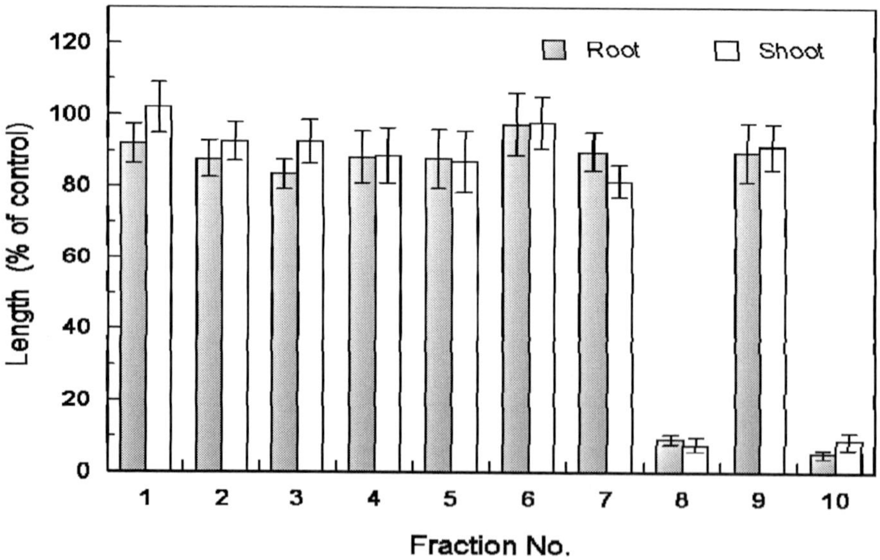

Figure 3. Effects of fractions obtained after column chromatography of ethyl acetate fraction isolated from an aqueous methanol extract of cucumber plant wastes. Root and shoots length of the cress seedlings was determined after 48 h of incubation in the dark at 25 °C. Fraction 1 (eluted by 20 % ethyl acetate in *n*-hexane), 2 (30 % ethyl acetate in *n*-hexane), 3 (40 % ethyl acetate in *n*-hexane), 4 (50 % ethyl acetate in *n*-hexane), 5 (60 % ethyl acetate in *n*-hexane), 7 (70 % ethyl acetate in *n*-hexane), 8 (80 % ethyl acetate in *n*-hexane), 9 (ethyl acetate) and 10 (methanol). Other detail as for Figure 1.

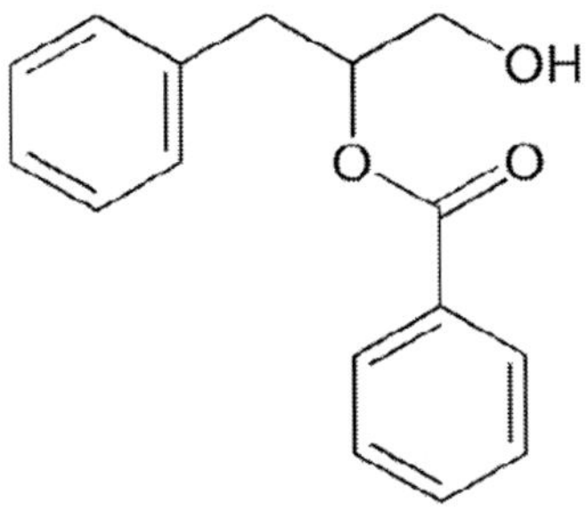

Figure 4. Chemical structure of (*S*)-2-benzoyloxy-3-phenyl-1-propanol.

Identification of Allelopathic Substance 1 and Biological Activity

The ^{1}H NMR (CD_3OD, 400 MHz, TMS as internal standard) spectrum of the substance **1** showed; δ 2.85 (1H, dd, *J*=13.7, 8.3 Hz), 3.02 (1H, dd, *J*=13.7, 6.3 Hz), 3.64 (2H, d, *J*=5.4 Hz), 4.33 (1H, m), 7.16 (1H, tt, *J*=8.8, 1.8 Hz), 7.26 (4H, m), 7.41 (2H, dd, *J*=7.4, 7.4 Hz), 7.49 (1H, tt, *J*=7.4, 1.5 Hz) and 7.72 ppm (2H, dd, *J*= 7.4, 1.5 Hz). The specific rotation of the substance was $[\alpha]_D^{24}$ -65.8° (c=0.087, MeOH). From the comparison of these data with those reported in the literature (Yaoita and Kikuchi, 1997), the substance was identified as (*S*)-2-benzoyloxy-3-phenyl-1-propanol (Figure 4). This substance was first isolated from *Petasites japonicus* as a new phenylpropanoid by Yaoita and Kikuchi (1997). However, it has not been reported so far that (*S*)-2-benzoyloxy-3-phenyl-1-propanol has growth inhibitory activity.

The biological activity of (*S*)-2-benzoyloxy-3-phenyl-1-propanol was determined with cress and *E. crus-galli* seedlings (Figure 5). At concentration greater than 10 μM, the substance inhibited the growth of the roots and shoots of cress and *E. crus-galli.* The concentrations required for 50 % inhibition of the cress roots and shoots in the assay (defined as I_{50}), as determined by a logistic regression analysis, was 21 and 23 μM, respectively, and I_{50} values of *E. crus-galli* roots and shoots were 164 and 142 μM, respectively.

Identification of Allelopathic Substance 2 and Biological Activity

The ^{1}H NMR ($CDCl_3$, 400 MHz, TMS as internal standard) spectrum of inhibitor **2** showed; δ: 0.94 (3H, s), 1.01 (3H, s), 1.28 (3H, d, *J*=6.3 Hz), 1.88 (3H, d, *J*=1.2 Hz), 2.07 (1H, d, *J*=17.1 Hz), 2.32 (1H, d, *J*=17.1 Hz), 2.50 (1H, d, *J*=9.3 Hz), 4.33 (1H, m), 5.52 (1H, dd, *J*=15.1, 9.3 Hz), 5.66 (1H, dd, *J*=15.1, 5.9 Hz) and 5.88 (1H, s). The optical rotation of the substance was $[\alpha]^{25}_D$= 217 (c=0.01, CH_2Cl_2). From the comparison of these data with those reported in the literature (Pabst et al. 1992; D'Abrosca et al. 2004), the substance was identified as 9-hydroxy-4,7-megastigmadien-9-one (3-oxo-α-ionol; Figure 6). 9-Hydroxy-4,7-megastigmadien-9-one was identified as the aglycone of a glucoside isolated from *Rubus idaeus* (Pabst et al., 1992) and reported to act as an insect attractant (Isida et al., 2008).

However, it has not been reported so far that 9-hydroxy-4,7-megastigmadien-9-one is a potent allelopathic substance in cucumber plants.

The biological activities of 9-hydroxy-4,7-megastigmadien-9-one and were determined with cress and *E. crus-galli* seedlings (Figure 7). 9-Hydroxy-4,7-megastigmadien-9-one inhibited the growth of cress roots and shoots at concentration greater than 0.3 μM, and inhibited thc growth of *E. crus-galli* roots and shoots at concentrations greater than 1 μM. I_{50} values of the cress roots and shoots in the assay, as determined by a logistic regression analysis, were 6.7 and 2.4 μM, respectively, and I_{50} values of *E. crus-galli* roots and shoots were 9.1 and 29.3 μM, respectively.

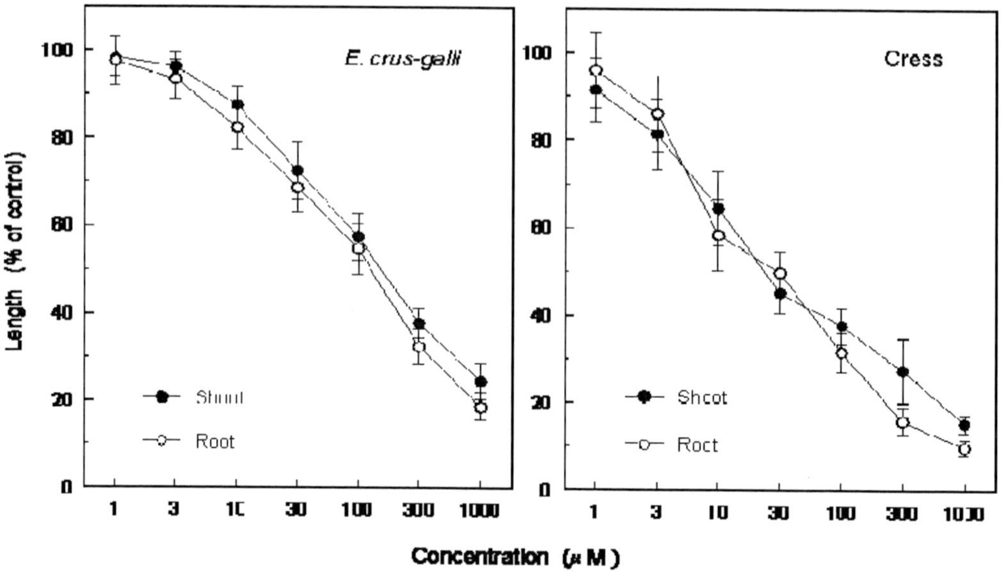

Figure 5. Effects of (*S*)-2-benzoyloxy-3- phenyl-1-propanol on the root and shoot growth of cress seedlings. Sample was dissolved in methanol, and added to two sheets of filter paper in a Petri dish. After germination, 10 seeds of cress or *Echinochloa crus-galli* were transferred to the Petri dish. Means ± SE from 5 independent experiments with 10 plants for each determination are shown. Other details as for Figure 1.

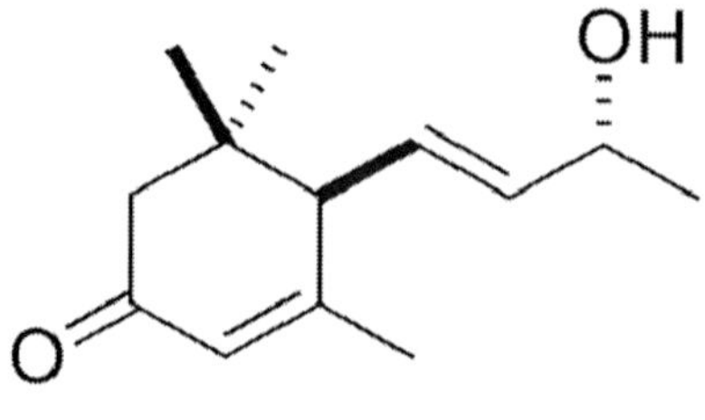

Figure 6. Chemical structure of 9-hydroxy-4,7-megastigmadien-9-one.

Identification of Active Substance 3 and Its Biological Activity

Fraction 10 by a silica gel column chromatography (Figure 3) was further purified Sephadex LH-20, C_{18} Sep-Pak cartridges, and HPLC, and an active substance **3** was isolated as colorless oil. Mass spectrum (FAB) of inhibitor **3** gave positive-mode molecular ion peak $[M+H]^+$ at *m/z* 241, suggesting a molecular weight of 240. The ^1H NMR (CD_3OD, 400 MHz, TMS as internal standard) spectrum of the substance showed; δ 5.89 (dd, *J* = 15.6, 1.0 Hz, 1H), 5.87 (s, 1H), 5.79 (dd, *J* = 15.6, 5.4 Hz, 1H), 4.19 (m, 1H), 3.50 (dd, *J* = 11.2, 4.9 Hz, 1H), 3.45 (dd, *J* = 11.2, 6.8 Hz, 1H), 2.50 (d, *J* =17.1 Hz, 1H), 2.14 (d, *J* = 17.1 Hz, 1H), 1.92 (d, *J* = 1.0 Hz, 3H).

The optical rotation of the substance was $[\alpha]_D^{25}$ +74.7° (c=0.13, MeOH). From the comparison of these data with those reported in the literature (Kai et al., 2007), the substance was identified as (6*S*,7*E*,9*S*)-6,9,10-trihydroxy-4,7-megastigmadien-3-one (Figure 8). This substance was recently isolated from cucumber as a new megastigmane (Kai et al., 2007). However, it has not been reported so far that (6*S*,7*E*,9*S*)-6,9,10-trihydroxy-4,7-megastigmadien-3-one has growth inhibitory activity.

(6*S*,7*E*,9*S*)-6,9,10-Trihydroxy-4,7-megastigmadien-3-one inhibited the growth of cress roots and shoots at concentration greater than 1 μM, and inhibited the growth of *E. crus-galli* roots and shoots at concentrations greater than 3 μM (Figure 9). I_{50} values of the cress roots and shoots in the assay, as determined by a logistic regression analysis, were 27.2 and 8.1 μM, respectively, and I_{50} values of *E. crus-galli* roots and shoots were 14.2 and 52.2 μM, respectively.

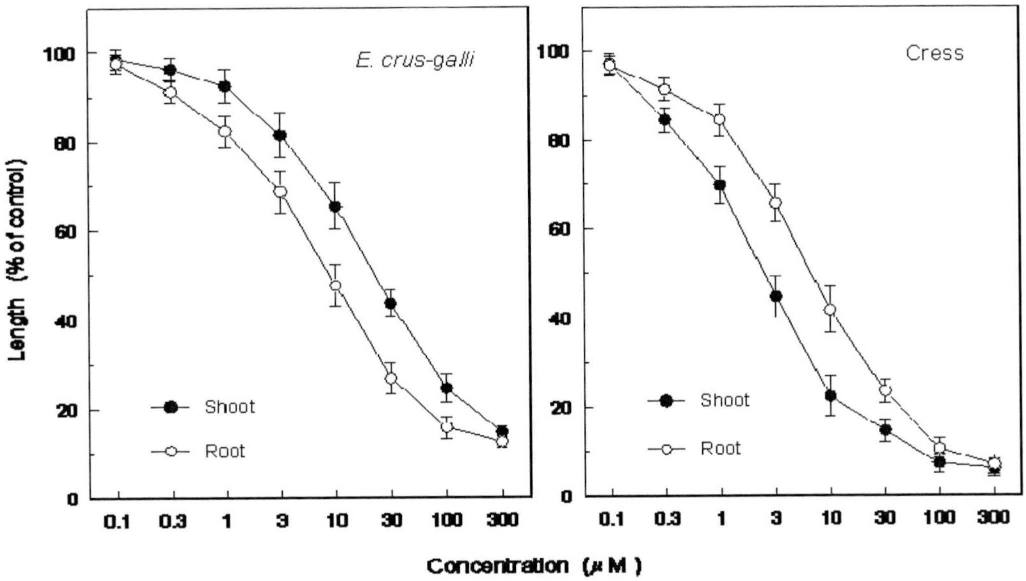

Figure 7. Effects of 9-hydroxy-4,7-megastigmadien-9-one on the root and shoot growth of cress and *Echinochloa crus-galli* (Kato-Noguchi et al., 2011). Other details as for Figures 1 and 5.

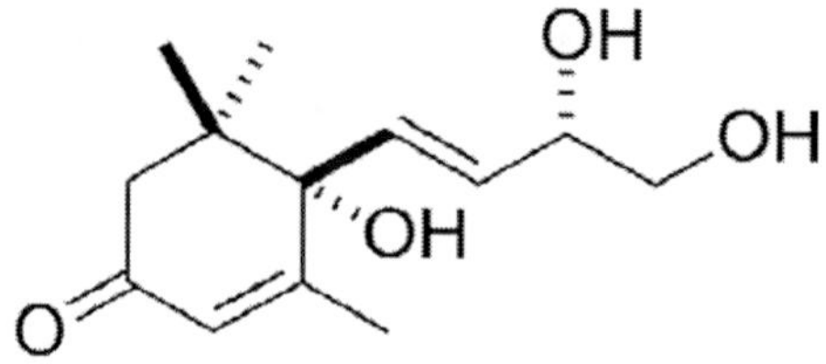

Figure 8. Chemical structure of (6*S*,7*E*,9*S*)-6,9,10-trihydroxy-4,7-megastigmadien-3-one.

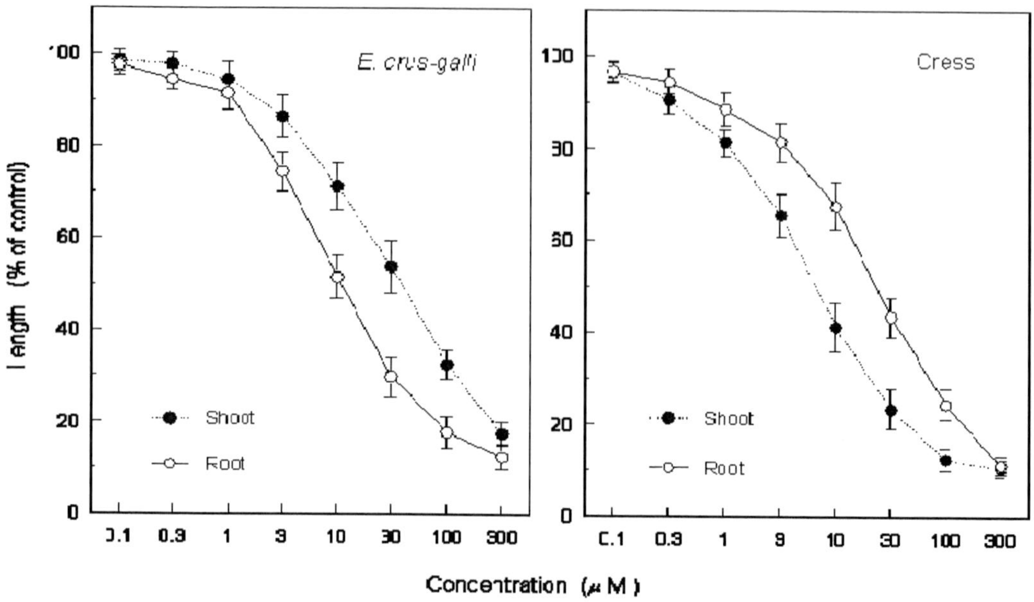

Figure 9. Effects of (6*S*,7*E*,9*S*)-6,9,10-trihydroxy-4,7-megastigmadien-3-one on the root and shoot growth of cress and *Echinochloa crus-galli* seedlings (Kato-Noguchi et al., 2011). Other details as for Figure 1 and 5.

Concentrations of Allelopathic Substances in Cucumber Plants

Concentrations of the allelopathic substances in cucumber plants were determined as described in Kato-Noguchi et al. (2011). The concentration of (*S*)-2-benzoyloxy-3-phenyl-1-propanol was the greatest and followed by (6*S*,7*E*,9*S*)-6,9,10-trihydroxy-4,7-megastigmadien-3-one and 9-hydroxy-4,7-megastigmadien-9-one (Table 4). Comparing I_{50} values, however, the inhibitory activity of 9-hydroxy-4,7-megastigmadien-9-one was the greatest and followed by (6*S*,7*E*,9*S*)-6,9,10-trihydroxy-4,7-megastigmadien-3-one and (*S*)-2-benzoyloxy-3-phenyl-1-propanol (Table 5).

If these compounds are released from 1 kg cucumber to 1 L soil water of the field either by exudates or decomposition of the plants, the concentration of (*S*)-2-benzoyloxy-3-phenyl-1-propanol (MW 256), 9-hydroxy-4,7-megastigmadien-9-one (MW 208) and (6*S*,7*E*,9*S*)-

6,9,10-trihydroxy-4,7-megastigmadien-3-one (MW 240) would be 290, 152 and 206 μM, respectively, based on the endogenous level (Table 4).

Table 4. Concentrations of active substances in cucumber wastes

Active substance	Concentration (mg/kg dry weight)
(*S*)-2-Benzoyloxy-3-phenyl-1-propanol	74.3 ± 7.2
9-Hydroxy-4,7-megastigmadien-9-one	31.8 ± 0.6
(6*S*,7*E*,9*S*)-6,9,10-Trihydroxy-4,7-megastigmadien-3-one	43.5 ± 0.4

Means ± SE from 5 independent experiments with three quantifications for each experiments are shown.

Table 5. I_{50} (μM) values of active substances

	Cress		*E. crus-galli*	
	Root	Shoot	Root	Shoot
(S)-2-Benzoyloxy-3-phenyl-1-propanol	21	23	164	142
9-Hydroxy-4,7-megastigmadien-9-one	6.7	2.4	9.1	29.3
(6S,7E,9S)-6,9,10-Trihydroxy-4,7-megastigmadien-3-one	27.2	8.1	14.2	52.2

I_{50} value is the concentrations required for 50 % inhibition of test plants in the assay and determined by a logistic regression analysis.

The threshold of 9-hydroxy-4,7-megastigmadien-9-one and (6*S*,7*E*,9*S*)-6,9,10-trihydroxy-4,7-megastigmadien-3-one, respectively, for growth inhibition was 10, 0.3 and 1 μM (Figures 5, 7 and 9). The estimated concentrations of both inhibitors in the soil water are over the threshold for the growth inhibition. Therefore, these substances may work as allelochemicals of cucumber plants.

ALLELOPATHY OF CUCUMBER

Many attempts have been made to exploit allelopathy of plants for weed control in a variety of agricultural settings (Inderjit, 1996; Seigler, 1996; Duke et al., 2000). It has been observed that some plant species can provide excellent weed suppression after incorporation of their residues into soil (Narwal, 1999; Semidey, 1999; Caamal-Maldoado et al., 2001). Plants produce hundreds of secondary compounds, and some of these compounds play an important role in allelopathy (Putnam, 1988; Gross and Parthier, 1994; Inderjit, 1996; Duke et al., 2000).

Powder of cucumber plants inhibited the growth of *E. crus-galli* (Table 3). Aqueous extracts and aqueous methanol extracts of cucumber plants inhibited the growth of all species tested (Table 1, Figure 1), which indicates that cucumber plants may have allelopathic substances. Three allelopathic substances were isolated from the aqueous methanol extract of cucumber plants and their chemical structures were determined as (*S*)-2-benzoyloxy-3-

phenyl-1-propanol, 9-hydroxy-4,7-megastigmadien-9-one and (6*S*,7*E*,9*S*)-6,9,10-trihydroxy-4,7-megastigmadien-3-one. These substances were active at concentrations greater than 0.3 - 10 μM (Figure 4, 7 and 9). Their levels in cucumber plants were 32 - 74 μg/kg cucumber plants (Table 4). Considering the endogenous level and the inhibitory activity, these substances may play important roles in the allelopathy of cucumber plants (Thi et al. 2008b; Kato-Noguchi et al., 2011). Under the certain conditions allelopathic substances are probably released into the plant rhizosphere, either as exudates from living tissues or by decomposition of plant residues in sufficient quantities to inhibit the growth of neighboring plants (Rice, 1984; Putnam, and Tang, 1986; Seigler, 1996; Einhellig, 1999; Belz, 2007). Therefore, allelopathic substances found in the cucumber plants research may provide the competitive advantage for root establishment of cucumber in the rhizosphere as allelochemicals which are involved in the defense mechanism through the inhibition of the growth of neighboring plant species that can be competitive with cucumber plants.

The negative impacts of commercial herbicide use on the environment make it desirable to diversify weed management options (Putnam, 1988; Weston, 1996; Einhellig, 1999; Tesio and Ferrero, 2010). Synthetic chemical herbicides may continue to be a key component in many integrated weed management systems, but controlling weeds through allelopathy is one strategy to reduce herbicide dependency (Putnam, 1988; Einhellig, 1996; Weston, 1996; Duke et al., 2000; Macías et al., 2007). Controlling weeds through cucumber allelopathy is one strategy to reduce dependency on the commercial herbicide. These biological active substances of the cucumber plants may work as weed suppressive agents.

Conclusion

It was found that cucumber plants have allelopathic potential and three allelopathic substances were isolated from the aqueous methanol extract of the cucumber plants harvested after crop production. The growth inhibitory activities of these substances are strong enough to cause growth inhibition of test plant species. Allelopathy may represent a new frontier for the implementation of the practices applicable in the sustainable weed management strategies. Another important approach is the identification of genes with allelopathic activities, and the application of breeding and transgenic techniques to place allelopathic traits into useful crop. In addition, allelochemicals have potential as either herbicides or templates for new herbicide classes because of strong herbicidal potential (Duke, 1986; Dodge 1987; Putnam, 1988; Gross and Parthier, 1994; Seigler, 1996; Duke et al., 2000; Macías et al., 2007).

References

Aburjai, T. and Natsheh, F.M. (2003) Plants used in cosmetics. *Phytotherapy Res.* 17, 987-1000.

Bais, H.P., Weir, T.L., Perry, L.G., Gilroy, S. and Vivanco, J.M. (2006) The role of root exudates in rhizosphere interactions with plants and other organisms. *Annu. Rev. Plant Biol.* 57, 233-266.

Belz, R.G. (2007) Allelopathy in crop/weed interactions - an update. *Pest. Manag. Sci.* 63, 308-326.

Caamal-Maldonado, J.A., Jiménez-Osornio, J.J., Torres-Barragán, A. and Anaya, A.L. (2001) The use of allelopahic legume cover and mulch species for weed control in cropping systems. *Agron. J.* 93, 25-27.

Chin, D.V. (2001) Biology and management of barnyarndgrass, red sprangletop and weedy rice. *Weed Biol. Manag.* 1, 37-41.

D'Abrosca, B., DellaGreca, M., Fiorentino, A., Monaco, P., Oriano, P. and Temussi, F., 2004. Structure elucidation and phytotoxicity of C_{13} *nor*-isoprenoids from *Cestrum parqui. Phytochemistry* 65, 497-505.

Dayan, F.E., Romagni, J.G. and Duke, S.O. (2000) Investigating the mode of action of natural phytotoxins. *J. Chem. Ecol.* 26, 2079-2094.

Duke, S.O. (1986) Naturally occurring chemical compounds as herbicides. *Rev. Weed Sci.* 2, 17-65.

Duke, S.O., Dayan, F.E., Romagni, J.G. and Rimando, A.M. (2000) Natural products as sources of herbicide, current status and future trends. *Weed Res.* 40, 99-111.

Dodge, A.D. (1987) Potential new targets for herbicides. *Pesti. Sci.* 20, 301-313.

Einhellig, F.A. (1999) An integrated view of allelochemicals amid multiple stresses. In: Inderjit., Dakshini, K.M.M., Foy, C.L. (Eds.). *Principals and Practices in Plant Ecology: Allelochemical Interactions*, CRC Press, Boca Raton, Florida, pp 479-494.

Gross, D. and Parthier, B. (1994) Novel natural substances acting in plant growth regulation. *J. Plant Grow. Regul.* 13, 93-114.

Hawes, M,C., Gunawardena, U., Miyasaka, S. and Zhao, X. (2000) The role of root border cells in plant defense. *Trends Plant Sci.* 5, 128-133.

Inderjit. (1996) Plant phenolics in allelopathy. *Bot. Rev.* 62, 186-202.

Ishida, T., Enomoto, H. and Nishida, R. (2008) New attractants for males of the solanaceous fruit fly *Bactrocera latifrons. J. Chem. Ecol.* 34, 1532-1535.

Jamir, T.T, Sharma, H.K. and Dolui, A.K. (1999) Folklore medicinal plants of Nagaland, India. *Fitoterapia* 70, 395-401.

Kai, H., Baba, M. and Okuyama, T. (2007) Two new megastigmanes from the leaves of *Cucumis sativus. Chem. Pharm. Bull.* 55, 133-136.

Kato-Noguchi, H., Thi, H.L., Teruya, T. and Suenaga, K. (2011) Two potent allelopathic substances in cucumber plants. *Sci. Hort.* (in press)

Macías, F.A., Molinillo, J.M.G., Varela, R.M. and Galindo, J.G.G. (2007). Allelopathy –a natural alternative for weed control. *Pest. Manag. Sci.* 63, 327-348.

McCully, E. (1999) Roots in soil: unearthing the complexities of roots and their rhizospheres. *Annu. Rev. Plant Physiol. Plant Mol. Biol.* 50, 695-718.

Narwal, S.S., 1999. Allelopathy in weed management. In: Narwal, S.S. (Ed.) Allelopathy Update. Vol. 2. *Basic and Applied Aspects*, Science Publishers Inc, Enfield, New Hampshire, pp 203-254.

Pabst, A., Barrona, D., Sémonb, E. and Schreier, P. (1992) Two diastereomeric 3-oxo-α-ionol β-glucosides from raspberry fruit. *Phytochemistry* 31, 1649-1652.

Potter, J.D. and Steinmetz, K. (1996) Vegetables, fruit and phytoestrogens as preventive agents. *IARC Sci. Pub.* 139, 61-90.

Putnam, A.R. and Duke, S.O. (1974) Biological suppression of weeds: evidence for allelopathy in accessions of cucumber. *Science* 185, 370-372.

Putnam, A.R. and Tang, C.-S. (1986) *The Science of Allelopathy*. John Wiley and Sons, New York.

Putnam, A.R. (1988) Allelochemicals from plants as herbicides. *Weed Technol.* 2, 510-518.

Rice, E.L. (1984) *Allelopathy*. Second ed. Academic Press, Orlando.

Rizvi, S.J.H. and Rizvi, V. (1992) *Allelopathy: Basic and Applied Aspects*. Chapman and Hall. London.

Seigler, D.S. (1996) Chemistry and mechanisms of allelopathic interactions. *Agron. J.* 88, 876-885

Semidey, N. (1999) Allelopathic crops for weed management in cropping systems. In: Narwal, S.S., (Ed.) *Allelopathy Update*. Vol. 2. Basic and Applied Aspects, Science Publishers Inc, Enfield, New Hampshire, pp 271-281.

Tesio, F. and Ferrero, A. (2010) Allelopthy, a chance for sustainable weed management. *Inter. J. Sustain. Dev. World Ecol.* 17, 377-389.

Thi, H.L., Lan, P.T.P., Chin, D.V. and Kato-Noguchi, H. (2008a) Allelopathy potential of Cucumber (*Cucumis Sativus*) on *Echinochloa crus-galli*. *Weed. Biol. Manag.* 9, 129-132.

Thi, H.L., Teruya, T., Suenaga, K., Chin, D.V. and Kato-Noguchi, H. (2008b) Allelopathy and the allelopathic activity of a phenylpropanol from cucumber plants. *Plant Grow. Regul.* 56, 1-5.

Xuan, T.D., Chung, I.M., Khanh, T.D. and Tawata, S. (2006) Identification of Phytotoxic substances from early growth of barnyard grass (*Echinochloa crus-galli*) root exudates. *J. Chem. Ecol.* 32, 895-906.

Weston, L.A. (1996) Utilization of allelopathy for weed management in agroecosystems. *Agron. J.* 88, 860-866.

Yaoita, Y. and Kikuchi, M. (1997) New phenylpropanoid and new eremophilenoides from rhizomes of *Petasites japonicus Maxim. Nat. Med.* 51, 372-375.

Yu, J.Q. and Matusi, Y. (1994) Phytotoxic substances in root exudates of cucumber (*Cucumis sativus* L.). *J. Chem. Ecol.* 20, 21-31.

Yu, J.Q., Sufeng, Y., Minh, F.Z. and Wen, H.H. (2003) Effects of root exudates and aqueous root extracts of cucumber (*Cucumis sativus*) and allelochemicals on photosynthesis and anti-oxidize enzymes in cucumber. *J. Biochem. System. Ecol.* 31, 129-131.

In: Vegetable Consumption and Health: New Research
Editors: Claudia Wilson and Melinda Morree
ISBN: 978-1-62100-941-2

Chapter 8

NITROGEN NUTRITION AND AMINO ACID METABOLISM IN CUCUMBER

***Ryota Tanemura*[1] *and Takuji Ohyama*[2]**
[1]Niigata Agricultural Research Institute, Horticultural Research Center, Japan
[2]Faculty of Agriculture, Niigata University, Japan

ABSTRACT

The characteristics of nitrogen nutrition and amino acid metabolism of cucumber plants were reviewed in relation to the nutritional values of fruits.

The water content in cucumber fruits is high at about 95% based on the fresh weight. They contain organic compounds, such as sugars, proteins, vitamins, fibers and amino acids and inorganic minerals such as potassium. The major free amino acids in cucumber fruits were glutamine and citrulline, with alanine, serine and glycine at lower levels. The fruits of Gourd family (*Cucurbitaceae*) contain relatively large amount of citrulline, which is known to improve a human blood flow. In anthesis of female flower, citrulline was already present in the ovary, and its content increased with the growth of fruit. The most part of absorbed nitrogen (about 90%) was translocated from roots to the aerial parts though xylem vessels in the form of nitrate (NO_3^-). Thus the most part of NO_3^- was reduced to amino acids mainly in the leaves. However, a small part of the absorbed nitrogen was also reduced in the roots and subsequently translocated to the aerial parts as amino acids such as glutamine and citrulline. In leaves, citrulline accumulation occurred and it was the dominant free amino acids. Accumulation of ammonium in leaves was not observed possibly due to its toxicity.

The absorbed nitrogen in the early stage of harvest was translocated rapidly to the leaves and assimilated there, then, the nitrogen in the leaves was retranslocated preferentially to the growing fruits. Based on ^{15}N analysis, approximately 50% of nitrogen contained in the harvested fruit was that absorbed after flowering of the fruit. Nitrogen absorbed before the harvest was also utilized in the formation of secondary lateral branches during fruit harevest period.

INTRODUCTION

Cucumber (*Cucumis sativus* L.) is thought to have been cultivated over 3,000 years, and is one of the most popular vegetables all over the world nowadays. The cucumber fruits are used not only as fresh vegetables, for example, in salads, but also as pickling and cooking materials. In 2006, the production of the cucumber in the world was about 44 million tons. China produced more than a half of the world production, and high production countries were recorded in Turkey, Iran, Russia, the United States, Ukraine, and Japan.

Because cucumber fruits contain a lot of water and the concentration of nutritive components in cucumber is relatively lower than that of other vegetables. The quality of cucumber fruits is usually classified based on the shape, uniformity, skin color and defects. In Japan, the cucumber fruits are harvested at immature stage based on fruit length (about 20cm) and fruit weight (about 100g) as a commercial standard size.

Recently, consumers are becoming more interested in their health, and there is a growing interest in minerals and amino acids compositions in cucumber fruits. The water content in cucumber fruits is high at about 95% of the fresh weight (Table1). They contain organic compounds, such as vitamins, sugars, proteins, fibers and amino acids and inorganic minerals (Table1). Among minerals, the cucumber fruits contain a lot of potassium, which has diuretic effect for human. The fruits of Gourd family (*Cucurbitaceae*) contain relatively a large amount of citrulline (Cit). Cit is one of the amino acids to have the effect on increasing the production of nitric oxide (NO). It is known that NO works to expand the blood vessels to increase human blood flow. By increasing blood flow, metabolism, fatigue, and cold constitution can be improved. The amino acid such as Cit is an organic compound consisting of carboxyl and amino groups. Therefore, the control of cultivation to accelerate the efficient photosynthesis and nitrogen nutrition and transport of C and N to the fruits is important to produce high-quality fruits which contain high concentration of Cit.

One of the characteristics of cucumber growth is that vegetative growth and reproductive growth proceed at the same time for a long period (several months) after initial flowering. The plant vigor of the cucumber is affected by temperature, humidity, irrigation, fertilization and stem training. It is very important to maintain a proper balance of vegetative growth and reproductive growth during the harvest period to maximize the fruits yield by pinching the stem buds and by controlling nutrient supply. The nitrogen-fixing plants such as leguminous plant can use nitrogen gas in the air, but only combined nitrogen is used by absorption from the root in most plants. Therefore, nitrogen fertilization is very important for controlling plant growth, vigor, as well as photosynthetic activity. Cucumber plants continue to produce new branches, new flowers and new fruits simultaneously for several months. Therefore, nitrogen supply may be necessary during the fruits harvest period. However, an excess amount of nitrogen fertilizer causes salt accumulation in the medium, resulting in poor fruit quality and decreases in the commercial yield. In addition, excess fertilization causes groundwater contamination by nitrate and phosphorus, and it will cause the emission of nitrous oxide (N_2O), which is a global warming gas (Miyazaki 2000; Noda 2001; Yoh and Minami 1991).

Recently, consumers and growers have been seeking environmentally friendly agriculture, where proper levels, forms and timing of fertilization are very important. To optimize the fertilizer rate from the viewpoint of high quality, low cost, saving labor and resources, and avoiding salt accumulation, it is necessary to investigate the characteristics of absorption and transport of supplied nitrogen in cucumbers.

This review focused on the characteristics of nitrogen nutrition and amino acid metabolism of cucumber plants.

Table 1. Concentration of nutrients in cucumber fruits (Per 100g fresh weight)

	Fresh fruits	Salted fruits	Pickled fruits (sweet)	Pickled fruits (sour)
Energy (kcal)	14	16	67	12
Water (g)	95.4	92.1	80	93.4
Protein (g)	1	1	0.3	1.4
Lipid (g)	0.1	0.1	0.1	0
Carbohydrate(g)	3	3.7	18.3	2.5
Ash (g)	0.5	3.1	1.3	2.7
Minerals				
Na (mg)	1	1000	440	1000
K (mg)	200	220	18	11
Ca (mg)	26	26	25	23
Mg (mg)	15	15	6	24
P (mg)	36	38	16	5
Fe (mg)	0.3	0.2	0.3	1.2
Zn (mg)	0.2	0.2	0.1	0.1
Cu (mg)	0.11	0.07	0.04	0.04
Mn (mg)	0.07	0.07	0	0.2
NaCl equivalent (g)	0	2.5	1.1	2.5
Vitamine				
A: β-carotene equivalent (μg)	330	210	53	14
A: Retinol equivalent (μg)	28	18	4	1
B1 (mg)	0.03	0.02	0	0.02
B2 (mg)	0.03	0.03	0.01	0.06
Niacin (mg)	0.2	0.2	0.1	0.1
B6 (mg)	0.05	0.06	0.04	0
B12 (μg)	0	0	0	0
Folic acid (μg)	25	28	2	1
Pantothenic acid (mg)	0.33	0.34	0	0
C (mg)	14	11	0	0

From "2009 All Guide Standard Tables of Food Composition in Japan, Fifth revised and enlarged edition"

Salted fruits: Cucumber fruits are treated with salt or put into salt water.

Pickled fruits (sweet): Cumuber fruits are soaked into vinegar with spices and sugar.

Pickled fruits (sour): Cumuber fruits are soaked into salt water then fermentated by lactic acid fermentation.

1. AMINO ACID AND SUGAR OF THE CUCUMBER FRUITS

In Japan, cucumber fruits are harvested at an immature stage, when the fruit length is about 20 cm and the fruit weigh is about 100g. Number of days required from anthesis to harvest depends on the variety and growing conditions and vigor of the plants. As shown in Figure 1, 2 and 3, number of days required from anthesis to harvest was as short as 5 days under good nutritional and weather conditions in late August, while during low temperature seasons fruits harvest required more than 20 days after anthesis in late October. Length of the cucumber fruit increased slowly for the first time after flowering, and then the elongation rate became gradually faster (Figure 1). The fruit weight increased after flowering was also initially slow, but the weight was rapidly increased just before harvest (Figure 2).

In vegetables, the main components affecting their taste are free amino acids and sugars. The major free amino acids in cucumber fruits are Gln, Cit, alanine (Ala), serine (Ser), glycine (Gly), glutamic acid (Glu) and aspartic acid (Asp). The most abundant amino acid was Gln, accounting for more than 50% of total free amino acids in cucumber fruit (Nakamach et al. 2002). As shown in Figure 4, total free amino acid concentration of the cucumber fruits in late August was temporarily increased after anthesis, however it decreased with rapid enlargement of the fruits, showing the maximum level at 3 days after anthesis. On the other hand, the amino acid content per a fruit increased with fruit enlargement (Figure 5).

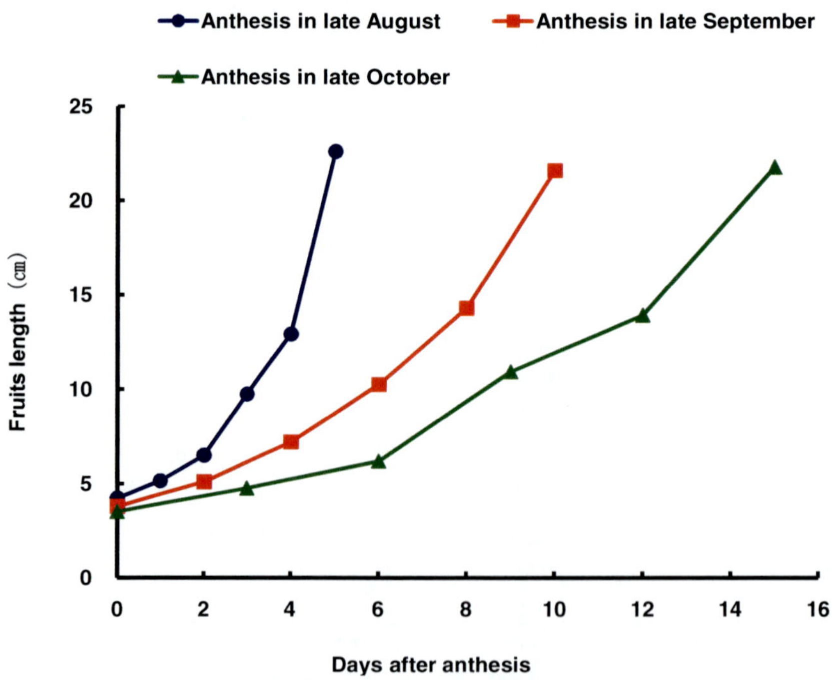

Figure 1. Effect of growth stage on the length of the cucumber fruits.

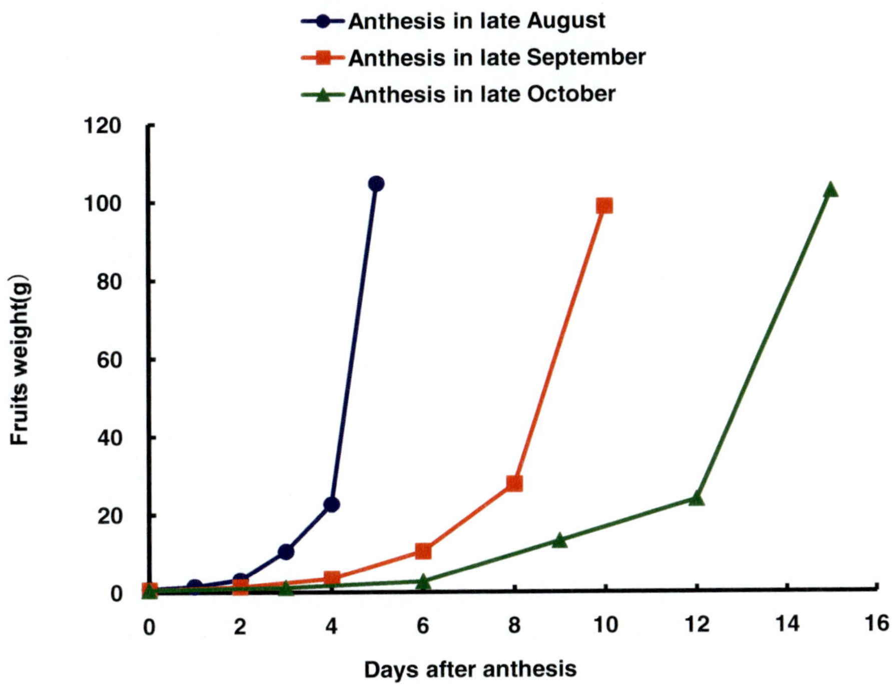

Figure 2. Effect of growth stage on the weight of the cucumber fruits.

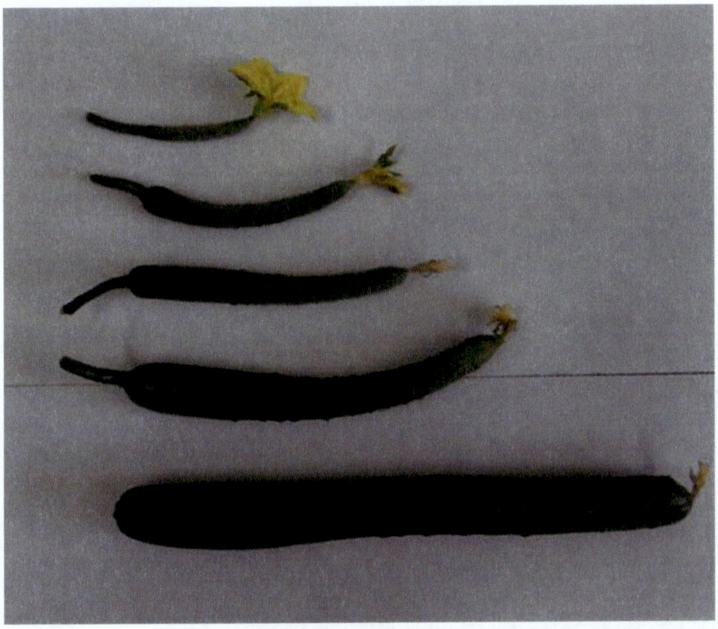

Figure 3. A photograph of enlargement process of cucumber fruits from anthesis (upper) to harvest (lower) in late August.

The fruits of Gourd family (*Cucurbitaceae*) contain relatively a large amount of Cit, which is known to improve a human blood flow. A level of Cit about 40% of total amino N are included in the cucumber fruits at the same level as Gln (Figure 6).

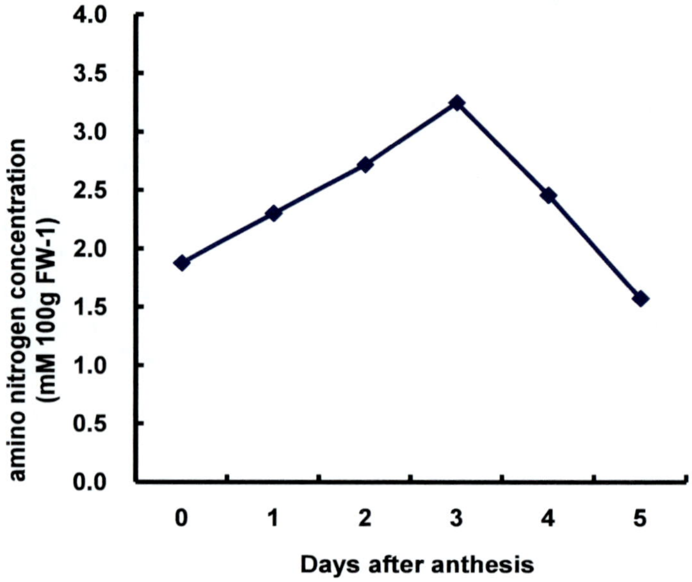

Figure 4. Changes in concentration of total free amino nitrogen in the cucumber fruits in late August.

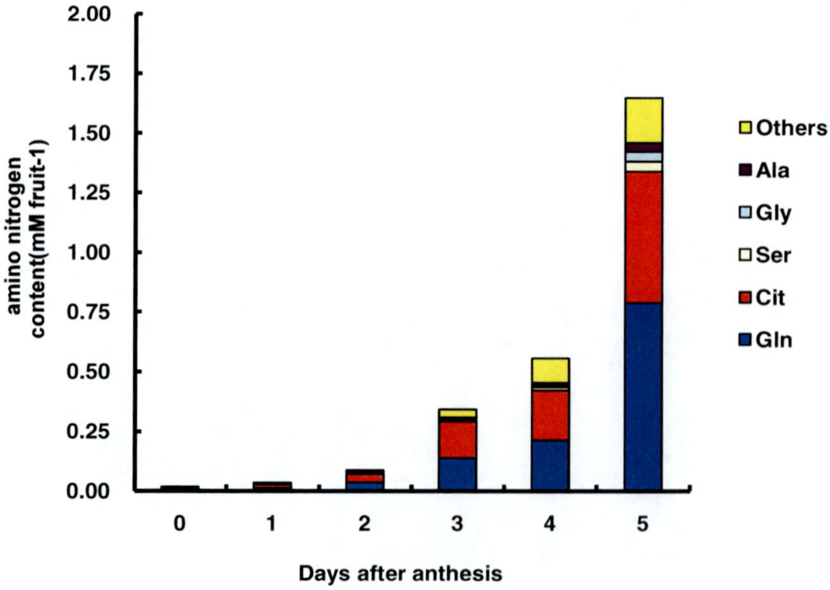

Figure 5.Changes in free amino nitrogen content in a cucumber fruit in late August.

In anthesis of female flower at day 0 (Figure 5, 6), Cit was already present in the ovary, and its content increased with the fruit enlargement. Recently, sweetness is a key factor for the taste quality and preference of cucumber. Sugar concentration of cucumber fruits is low just after anthesis, then increases with the enlargement of the fruits, especially fruits sugars accumulated rapidly just before harvest (Davies and Kempton 1976).

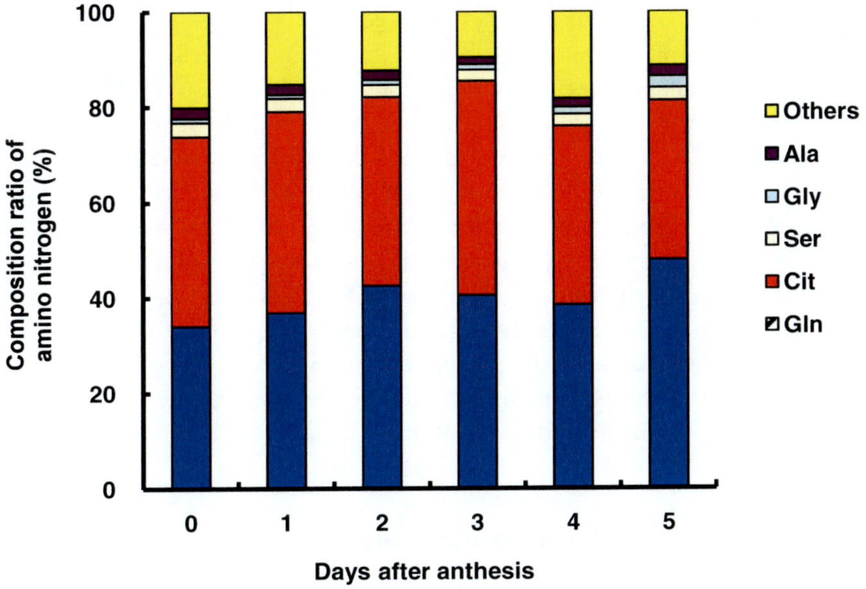

Figure 6. Changes in composition ratio of amino nitrogen of the cucumber fruits in late August.

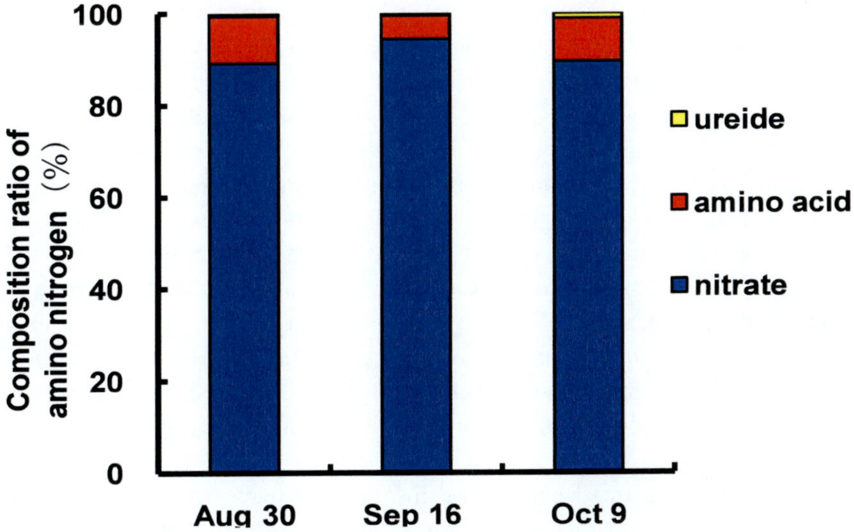

Figure 7. Changes in composition ratio of nitrogen of the cucumber xylem. September 16: Start of harverst, October 9: Peak of harvest.

Strength of sweetness is different depending on the kind of sugar, and the sweetness degree is high in fructose, sucrose, and glucose in this sequence. The main soluble sugars in cucumber fruits are glucose and fructose at nearly equal amounts, with extremely small amount of sucrose and others (Nakamach et al. 2002, Davies and Kempton 1976, Horie 2011).

Just before harvest stage the fruits rapidly enlarged, therefore, a large amount of photoassimilate supply during this period is required for increasing the sugar concentration in harvested fruits. On the other hand, sugar content is known to decrease when photoassimilate supply is not enough under defective weather conditions (Horie 2011). It is reported that a high-quality tomato fruits with a high sugar concentration could be produced by the salt stress and the water stress (Zushi et al. 2005, Saito et al. 2006). However, in the cucumber, the translocation of photoassimilate to the fruits was reduced by salinity in the medium, as a result, salinity decreased sugar concentrations in cucumber fruits and increased occurrence of bent fruits, and reduced fruits yield (Tazuke 2001, Kanahama and Saito 1988).

In plants, amino acid synthesis is performed by the use of photoassimilate synthesized by the leaves and absorbed inorganic nitrogen from roots. It is important that the balance of the reproductive growth and the vegetative growth is kept by proper nitrogen fertilization and an efficient translocation of the photoassimilates and the nitrogenous metabolites to cucumber fruits for high-quality cucumber fruits production.

2. Nitrogen Assimilation

The major forms of inorganic nitrogen, which plants can absorb, are NH_4^+-N and NO_3^--N. In the upland field, fertilized NH_4^+ is rapidly oxidized to NO_3^- by nitrifying bacteria in the soil. Therefore, a najor form of nitrogen absorbed by cucumber roots is NO_3^--N. The absorbed NO_3^- should be reduced to ammonia before it is assimilated into various organic compounds. Plants reduce absorbed nitrate into nitrite via nitrate reductase (NR; EC 1.6.6.1) and ammonium via nitrite reductase (NiR; EC 1.6.6.4) in roots and leaves. Ammonium (NH_4^+) is an initial material of the nitrogen assimilation in plants. However, NH_4^+ is toxic when it is accumulated in cells. Therefore, ammonium is usually rapidly assimilated into amino acids through the glutamine synthetase (GS; EC 6.3.1.2) and glutamate synthase (GOGAT; EC 1.4.1.14) pathway, and the plant doesn't usually accumulate ammonia at a high level. In plants, the nitrogen absorbed from the roots is translocated to the shoots as a NO_3^--N and amino acids. In the cucumber, the NR activity of the roots is lower than that of the leaves, and NO_3^- is reduced in the amino acid mainly in the leaves (Ouji and Hirata 1976, Tachibana et al. 1991). In our result, the most part (about 90%) of the absorbed nitrogen was translocated from the roots to the aerial parts in the form of NO_3^- from though xylem vessels irrespective of the stages (Figure 7).

On the other hand, a small part of the absorbed nitrogen was reduced in the roots and subsequently translocated to the aerial parts as in the form of amino acids. As shown in Figure 8, the amino acid compositions in the xylem sap were almost the same irrespective of the growth stages. The most abundant amino acid was Gln, which accounted for about 68-78% of the total amino nitrogen. In addition, Cit, arginine (Arg) and Asp contents were relatively high. Rice and barley assimilate the absorbed NH_4^+-N to asparagine (Asn), and it is accumulated in the roots and the leaves. Due to the activity, the tolerance to NH_4^+-N may be strong in these plants (Ouji and Izawa 1974a, Ouji and Izawa 1974b). In peanut and soybean, the most abundant amino acid in xylem sap was asparagine, which was about 40-80% of the total amino acids. (Goto et al. 1989, Inanaga and Inomoto 1994, Ohyama et al. 1994).

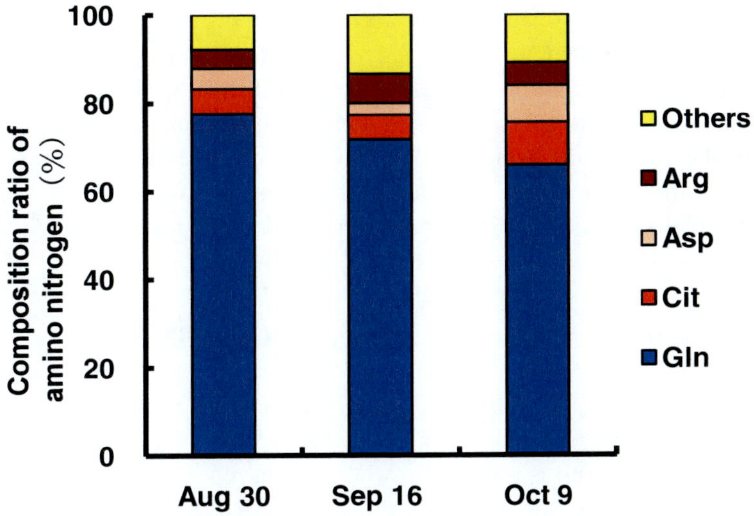

Figure 8. Changes in composition ratio of amino nitrogen of the cucumber xylem. September 16: Start of harverst, October 9: Peak of harvest.

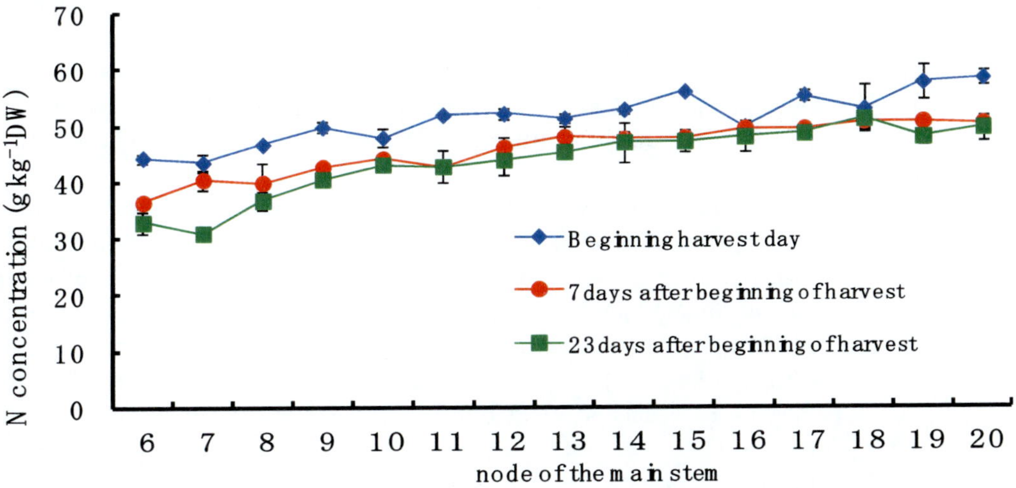

Figure 9. Changes in the nitrogen concentration in the leaves of the each node of the main stem. Bars denote the standard deviations (n = 3).

In contrast, Asn was not major amino acid in the xylem sap of cucumber. Therefore, when a cucumber absorbs NH_4^+-N in large quantities, the growth was inferior due to ammonium toxicity. Asn is synthesized from aspartic acid and Gln by asparagine synthetase (EC 6.3.5.4), and the Asp is synthesized from oxaloacetate and glutamate by aspartate aminotransferase (EC 2.6.1.1). On the other hand, Gln is synthesized from ammonium and glutamate by glutamine synthetase. Difference of the amino acid composition of xylem in rice and cucumber is considered to be different due to the balance of these plant enzyme activities (Ouji and Izawa 1974a, 1974b).

In cucumber, the most part of the absorbed nitrogen was translocated in the form of NO_3^- from roots to the leaves in xylem. However, little accumulation of NO_3^--N in the leaves was observed and the NO_3^- translocated to the leaves was reduced and metabolized rapidly. Furthermore, NH_4^+ didn't accumulate in the leaves, pssibly because NH_4^+ is immediately assimilated into amino acids. In cucumber leaves, a high accumulation of Cit occurred and it was shown that Cit is the main component of free amino acids in leaves. Reduction of NO_3^- to ammonia and Cit formation in cucumber fruits are closely related. Cit is accumulated in the leaves but it was metabolized rapidly by nitrogenous requirement of cucumber.

3. Absorption and Translocation

In cucumber, after harvest of fruits starts, many parts of the plant become sinks in addition to the fruits, for example, the female flowers and new leaves and branches. However, the sink strength of the specific fruit is especially strong during reproductive stage. Thus, the photoassimilate is translocated intensively to the fruits, and consequently, the translocation to other organs may decrease (Murakami et al 1982). Therefore, after the flowering period, the increase in dry weight of cucumber fruits is much higher than the increase in the other vegetable fruits, such as eggplants and strawberry (Tanemura et al. 2008, Takano and Suzuki 1989, Forney and Breen 1985). In cucumber, nitrogen absorbed before the harvest began was translocated to the new secondary lateral branches in the fruit enlargement term. It can be considered that the nitrogen absorbed in the vegetative growth phase is important in the occurrence of the lateral branch in the fruit enlargement term, and that the condition of nitrogen nutrition before the harvest influences the occurrence of the lateral branch (Tanemura et al. 2008).

The nitrogen concentrations of leaves and stems tended to decrease after the fruits harvest started (Yanai 1975, Tanemura et al. 2008). The nitrogen concentration tended to be higher in the upper leaves than the lower leaves and gradually decreased after beginning of harvest (Figure 9). The similar trend, that the nitrogen concentration of the leaves and stems decreased during the fruits growth stage, were reported in eggplant (Takano and Suzuki 1989), melon (Fukutoku et al. 2000) and green pepper (Uesugi and Fujita 1972). Therefore, the nitrogen in the leaves and stems is exported to a sink organ, especially growing fruits, in the cucumber plants as well.

The translocation rate of nitrogen from the leaves to the fruits is higher than the changes in the distribution rate of the dry matter in the fruit enlargement stage of the eggplant (Takano and Suzuki 1989). The 76% of nitrogen absorbed after pollination was distributed in the fruits of melon (Fukutoku et al. 2000). When the sink activity of the fruit increased, the assimilated nutrients were transported more preferentially to the fruits than to the vegetative organs in tomato (Heuvelink 1997; Heuvelink and Buiskool 1995). The increase rate of the nitrogen content of the cucumber fruits was higher than that of the dry matter, and the increase in the nitrogen content of the fruits accounted for 74% of the whole plant (Tanemura et al. 2008).

Furthermore, in the 7 days from the harvest-starting day, approximately 20% of nitrogen that existed in the organs except for the fruits was translocated to the fruits. During that period, the leaves of the main stem had the strongest translocation activity (source activity) of nitrogen compared with other organs, 23% of nitrogen contained in the leaves of the main stem translocated to other organs. This quantity was equivalent to approximately 70% of the amount of increases of nitrogen in the fruits. The nitrogen content of the leaves of the main stem was higher in the upper leaves than the lower leaves. The amount of nitrogen translocation to other organs was higher in the upper leaves than in the lower leaves. The assimilative capacity of these leaves declined markedly in comparison with the upper new leaves (Tanemura et al. 2008).

In the 7 days from the harvest-starting day, approximately 33% of nitrogen absorbed in the 7 days was distributed in the fruits. In the 16-day after that, approximately 41% of nitrogen was redistributed to fruits from leaves, stems and roots (Tanemura et al. 2008). The nitrogen assimilated into leaves near the fruit-set node is preferentially translocated to the fruit in melons (Fukutoku et al. 2000). In contrast, in the case of cucumber, fruits can receive photoassimilate from leaves that are located at a node far from the fruit-set node (Murakami et al. 1982).

A large amount of nitrogen was translocated from the upper young leaves, in which the assimilative capacity might be high (Tanemura et al. 2008). Therefore, fruits are strong sinks in fruit enlargement terms in cucumber, and all the vegetative organs, especially the leaves, are working as a source of nitrogen.

The nitrogen absorbed within 24 h before the harvest accounted for 6.1% of all nitrogen in the harvested fruits, and 50% of nitrogen contained in the harvest fruit of the cucumber is nitrogen absorbed after flowering (Tanemura et al. 2008). Some part of the absorbed nitrogen might be translocated rapidly to the fruits; however, most of the nitrogen was assimilated in the leaves and retranslocated to the fruits thereafter. The source–sink relationship of nitrogen is similar to that of the photoassimilate in melon (Fukutoku et al. 2000). Although fruit set is different in the melon and the cucumber, it can be considered that the source–sink relationship of the photoassimilate may be similar to the movement of nitrogen in the cucumber.

CONCLUSIONS

Cucumber plants prefer NO_3^- and high concentration of NH_4^+ is toxic. Most of the NO_3^- absorbed in the roots is transported to the shoot through xylem vessels, and reduced to NO_2^- by Nitrate reductase, then to NH_4^+ by Nitrite reductase in the leaves (Figure 10). Small part of NO_3^- is reduced and assimilated in the roots and transported to the shoot mainly in the form of glutamine. Leaves are the main source organ of N to the fruits. The major parts of free amino acids in cucumber fruits are glutamine and citrulline. Citrulline is considered to be a good for human health.

Cucumber fruits obtain about 50% of N from the N absorbed after anthesis, and the other 50% was from redistribution of N from leaves, stems and roots which assimilated the N before anthesis. Therefore, to produce cucumber fruits with high yield and good quality need sufficient supply of N not only before initial anthesis, but also during fruits harvesting stage.

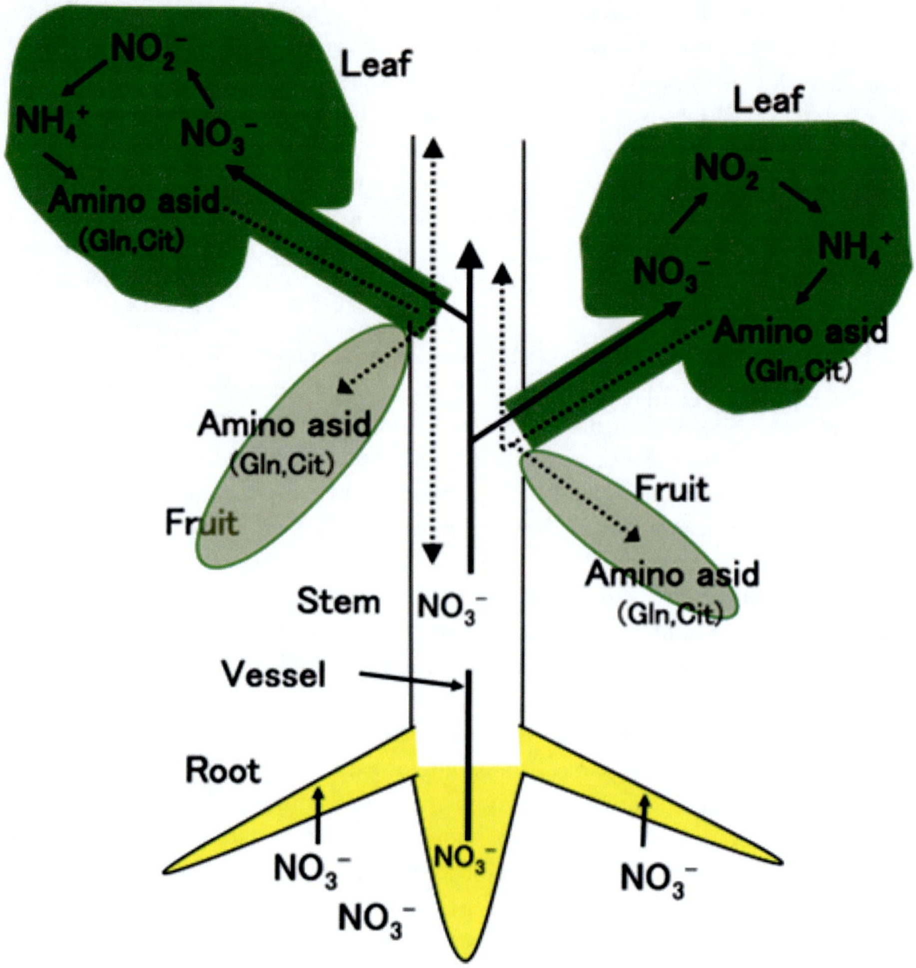

Figure 10. The model of the translocation of nitrogen in the cucumber.

References

[1] A*ll Guide: Standard Table of Food Composition in Japan* (2009) Fifth revised and enlarged edition, Jikkyo Shuppan Co., Ltd.

[2] Davies JN and Kempton RJ (1976) Some change in Composition of the Fruit of Glasshouse Cucumber (*Cucumis sativus*) during Growth, Maturation and Senescence. *J. Sci. Food Agric*., 27, 413-418.

[3] Forney CF and Breen PJ (1985) Dry matter partitioning and assimilation in fruiting and deblossomed strawberry. *J. Am. Soc. Hort. Sci*., 110, 181–185.

[4] Fukutoku Y, Teraoka Y, Koto S and Kubo K (2000) Nitrogen absorption and distribution of muskmelons (*Cucumis melo* L.) at different growth stages using hydroponics. *Jpn. J. Soil Sci. Plant Nutr*., 71, 72–81.

[5] Goto S, Inanaga S and Kumazawa K (1989) Xylem sap composition of nodulated and non-nodulated groundnut plants. *Soil Sci. Plant Nutr*. 33.619-627.

[6] Heuvelink E (1997) Effect of fruit load on dry matter partitioning in tomato. *Scientia Hortic.*, 69, 51–59.

[7] Kanahama K and Saito T (1988) Carbohydrate distribution and ^{14}C-photosynthates uptake in the curved fruits of cucumber. *Jpn. J. Soc. Hort. Sci.,* 57, 448–453.

[8] Heuvelink E and Buiskool RPM (1995) Influence of sink source interaction on dry matter production in tomato. *Ann. Bot.*, 75, 381–389.

[9] Horie H (2011) Day-to-Day Fluctuation of the Sugar Contebnts in Cucumber Fruits and the Application of Disposable Blood Glucose Sensors for Quality Estimation of the Fruits. *Hort. Res. Japan.* 10(1). 109-113.

[10] Inanaga S and Inomoto Y (1994) Translocating Form of N to Peanut Fruit. *Jpn. J. Soil Sci. Plant Nutr.*, 65, 554–559.

[11] Miyazaki N (2000) Studies on the actual and qualitative condition of underground water in the areas in southern Tochigi Prefecture that plant upland crops. *Bull. Tochigi Agr. Exp. Stn*, 49, 47–57.

[12] Murakami T, Inayama M and Kobayashi H (1982) Translocation and distribution of ^{14}C-photosynthates in cucumber plants. *Bull. Nat. Inst. Agr. Sci. Series D*, 33, 235–275.

[13] Nakamach A, Yoshikawa M, Kasai M and Hatae K (2002) Change and Distribution of Taste Components during the Storage of Cucumber. *Journal of Cookery Science of Japan*, 35(3), 234-241.

[14] Noda S (2001) Application and use of fertilizers for the reduction of nitrous oxide emissions from upland soils. *Jpn. J. Soc. Soil Sci. Plant Nutr.,* 72, 575–581.

[15] Ohyama T, Ohtake N, Nishiwaki T, Mizukoshi K, Minagawa R, Kobayashi K, Chinushi T and Takahashi Y (1994) Effect of N Fertilization on Seed Quality and Xylem Transport Form in Nodulating and Non-nodulating Soybean Isolines. *Bull. Facul. Agric. Niigata Univ.* 46. 57-70.

[16] Ouji Y, Izawa G (1974a) Studies on the Absorption and Assimilation of Inorganic Nitrogen in Intact Plants (Part 3). *Jpn. J. Soil Sci. Plant Nutr.*,45, 259-262.

[17] Ouji Y, Izawa G (1974b) Studies on the Absorption and Assimilation of Inorganic Nitrogen in Intact Plants (Part 4). *Jpn. J. Soil Sci. Plant Nutr.*,45, 341-351.

[18] Ouji Y, Hirata M (1976) Difference in Nitrate Reducing Ability of Rice and Cucumber Plants. *Jpn. J. Soil Sci. Plant Nutr.*,47, 178-182.

[19] Saito T, Fukuda N and Nishimura S (2006) Effects of Salinity Treatment Duration and Planting Density on Size and Sugar Content of Hydroponically Grown Tomato Fruits. *J.Japan.Soc. Hort. Sci.* 75(5). 392-398.

[20] Tachibana S, Konishi N, Kanda H (1991) Diurnal variation of in vivo and in vitro nitrate reductase activity in cucumber plants. *Jpn. J. Soc. Hort. Sci.,* 60, 593–599.

[21] Takano T, Suzuki K (1989) Changesin nutrient uptake rate and translocation of nutrients in the developmental stage of eggplant. *Sci. Rept Fac. Agr. Meijo Univ.*, 25, 17–25.

[22] Tanemura R, Kurashima Y, Ohtake N, Sueyoshi K and Ohyama T (2008) Absorption and translocation of nitrogen in cucumber (*Cucumis sativus* L.) plants using the ^{15}N tracer technique. *Soil Sci. Plant Nutr.*, 54, 108-117.

[23] Tazuke A (2001) Sugar Concentration of Cucumber Fruit as Affected by NaCl Addition to Nutrient Solution. *Environ. Control in Biol.* 39(4). 235-243.

[24] Uesugi I and Fujita Y (1972) Comparison the growth and nutrient absorption and yield of sweet pepper usually received heavy fertilizer with it received light fertilizer on sandy soil in vinyl house. *Bull. Kochi Inst. Agr. Forest Sci.,* 4, 1–8.

[25] Yanai T (1975) Effect of nitrogenous fertilizer on the growth of cucumber plants in relation to soil type and application method in a vinyl house. *Bull. Kochi Inst. Agr. Forest Sci.*, 7, 29–41.

[26] Yoh M and Minami K (1991) Emission of biogenic gas compounds from soil ecosystem and their effects on global environment. *Jpn. J. Soil Sci. Plant Nutr.,* 62, 654–661.

[27] Zushi K, Matsuzoe N, Yoshida S and Chikushi J (2005) Comparison of Chemical Composition Contents of Tomato Fruit grown under Water and Salinity Stresses. *J. SHITA*. 17(3). 128-136.

In: Vegetable Consumption and Health: New Research
Editors: Claudia Wilson and Melinda Morree
ISBN: 978-1-62100-941-2

Chapter 9

Safety Concerns Regarding Certain Herbs used on the Largest U.S. - Mexico Border

Armando González-Stuart*
University of Texas at El Paso, TX, U. S.

Abstract

Since the United States Congress passed the Dietary Supplements and Health Education Act (DSHEA) in October of 1994, an herbal product can be classified as a nutritional supplement. For this reason, many of the products bought as nutritional supplements may contain herbs in some form or another. The DSHEA encouraged the marketing of diverse herbal products including teas, extracts, essential oils, syrups, used both for healing, as well as aesthetic purposes. The United States and Mexico share a very extensive international border, and studies suggest that herbal product use is even more common along the border area, compared to the rest of the country. Some people are still under the impression that because herbal products are "natural", they are necessarily safe, and devoid of side effects. The lack of adequate quality control present in some herbal product companies around the world leads to variability in the quantity and quality of the products' content. Serious intoxications have occurred around the globe due to mislabeling of herbal products or erroneous identification of some plant species. Interactions between herbal products and certain prescription and over the counter (OTC) medications can sometimes be serious. Various herbal supplements which are new to the U.S. market have not been adequately tested for purity, safety or efficacy. This chapter presents information regarding the safety of selected medicinal herbs used on the U. S. -Mexico border. Due to the lack of reliable clinical data regarding the safe use of various herbal products currently available, it is imperative that the public be aware about the possible health hazard of using certain herbs for therapeutic purposes.

Keywords: Medicinal Plants, Toxicology, Herbal Safety, Herbal supplements, Complementary and Alternative Medicine

---

* asgonzalez1@utep.edu.

Introduction

Herbal medicine is the oldest form of healthcare known to mankind. Herbs have been used by all cultures throughout history and are an integral part of the development of modern civilization. From generation to generation, a wide array of herbal remedies have been employed in Mexico for the treatment of diverse ailments including gastrointestinal complaints, parasites (both external and internal), rashes, colds, diabetes and even cancer, to name just a few (Aguilar, 1999). Recently, however, the international market has been flooded by a legion of herbal products which may or may not be safe and effective. The purpose of this chapter is to mention some species of medicinal plants currently used in traditional medicine which could pose a hazard to health.

The Surge of Complementary and Alternative Medicine (CAM) in the United States

During the decade of the 1990's, the use of complementary and alternative medicine (CAM), including herbal supplements increased exponentially in the United States. The congressional act approving the Dietary Supplement and Health Education act (DSHEA) in October of 1994, facilitated the marketing of herbal and nutritional supplements classified as foods, not drugs. This made it easier for these products to be integrated into the mainstream market, available to the general public as over the counter products (OTC), not requiring a medical prescription (Dickinson, 2011).

While usage has increased, some information about the efficacy or safety of certain medicinal plants is either misleading, or simply unavailable. Some of these medicinal herbal products may indeed possess therapeutic value, but only if used properly and under the guidance of a professional.

Too often it is stated that herbal products are natural and therefore, safe. Unfortunately, this is not always the case, serious intoxications can occur due to mislabeling of herbal products or erroneous identification

Prevalence of Herbal Product Use in the Largest U. S. - Mexico Border Community

Research undertaken by the University of Texas at El Paso Pharmacy Program indicates that almost three quarters of the people living in the sister cities of Ciudad Juárez, Chihuahua, and El Paso, Texas, use diverse types of herbal products, both for medicinal as well as aesthetic purposes. Due to their popularity in Mexican traditional/folk medicine, the use of medicinal herbs along the largest border community in North America tends to be much higher compared to the rest of the United States (González-Stuart and Rivera, 2008).

Candle Nut Tree

This tree (*Aleurites moluccana* – Euphorbiaceae) is also known by the common names of: Indian walnut, Kukui, Tuitui, *Nuez de la India*, and *Palo de la India*

The tree is originally from Asia, but is now cultivated in South America, especially in Brazil. The fruits and leaves of this plant are used in traditional Asian medicine for the treatment of headache, morning sickness, fever, inflammation, gonorrhea, and to lower cholesterol (Pedrosa et al., 2002; Ostraff et al., 2000). Plant extracts showed anti-bacterial activity against *Staphylococcus aureus* and *Pseudomonas aeruginosa* (Locher et al., 1995).

The seeds have recently been touted as having various medicinal effects, but no controlled clinical trials have ever been undertaken in humans to evaluate their potential beneficial or toxicological effects.

Various ads claim the seeds of the plant can help in weight loss, as well as to lower cholesterol levels, although there are no known clinical studies to support these claims.

Some websites also mention the seed is useful for a plethora of conditions including arthritis, baldness, cellulite, constipation, hemorrhoids, to improve skin conditions, as an appetite suppressant, and as an aid to stop cravings for tobacco.

As aforementioned, there are no known clinical studies in humans to verify the various health claims made by some commercial companies which market candle nut tree seeds. Since the seeds can have a drastic purgative action (Wagstaff, 2008; Nelson et al., 2007; Hocking, 1997), they should not be used without supervision from a health professional, especially in patients with colitis (inflammation of the large intestine), or IBS (irritable bowel syndrome).

A woman was hospitalized in Navarra (Spain) after ingesting a candle nut seed product for weight loss. The patient showed hypotension, bradycardia, and was semi conscious. The patient had ingested potions of the seed many days prior to being admitted to the emergency room. (Pamplona, 2007).

Individuals suffering from any type of liver, heart or kidney disease should avoid ingesting the seed in any quantity.

Matarique

In Mexico this plant (*Psacalium decompositum* - Asteraceae) is also know but us common indigenous names of *Matariki*, and *Maturín*. These plants grow wild in semi- arid areas in northern Mexico, Arizona, and New Mexico.

The fresh root reputedly has great medicinal value for the treatment of various ailments. The root is boiled in water to make a tea. In Mexican traditional medicine, Matarique is used primarily against Type 2 diabetes, as well as for other gastrointestinal and urinary ailments.

Pyrrolizidine alkaloids have been detected in various species of the genus *Psacalium*, and are known to be liver toxic, as well as carcinogenic. Even though intoxications due to this plant have not been reported, Matarique has not been studied in depth in relation to its potential toxicity, especially with prolonged ingestion.

Do not consume teas or preparations made from this plant during prolonged periods of time (more than 2 weeks). Avoid ingesting this plant during pregnancy and lactation.

Mexican Arnica

This plant (*Heterotheca inuloides* - Asteraceae) is commonly known as False arnica, Telegraph plant, *Árnica mexicana*, and *Árnica del país*. This and other related species grow wild in many parts of Mexico and ther Southwestern United States. Various products containing this plant are available throughout Mexico, including some cities bordering the United States (Adame and Adame, 2000).

Products containing Mexican arnica can be ointments and lotions for external or topical application as well as teas, tablets, or homeopathic tinctures and pellets for internal use.

This plant has very similar uses to those of European Arnica (*Arnica montana* - Asteraceae) which is the species more commonly used both in Europe and the United States. Both European and Mexican arnica belong to the daisy or sunflower family, although their active principles are not identical.

Ointments and lotions made from this plant are used to treat bruises, sprains, rheumatism, varicose veins, and diverse skin infections due to bacteria and fungi (molds). The active ingredients in this plant have mild anti-inflammatory, analgesic, and antiseptic actions.

In Mexican traditional medicine, arnica teas have been taken internally for the treatment circulatory problems, nervous disorders, stomach ailments, and ulcers, as well as fever. Internal use of this plant is not recommended, due to its potential toxicity (Martinez, 1989).

Supplements containing arnica should be avoided internally during pregnancy and lactation. Arnica teas, tablets and other products containing this plant (or similar species, such as European arnica *Arnica montana*, for example), should not be taken internally, due to their potential toxicity, especially by small children, and patients suffering from heart disease. Both species of arnica may contain *helenalin*, a sesquiterpene compound that may interfere with normal blood clotting.

Homeopathic drops or pills containing Mexican arnica are usually diluted medications and may be safe to use, but should not be taken internally without the prior consent of a health professional. Do not apply arnica ointments, lotions, or pastes on broken skin, as this may cause irritation.

Wereke

The root of this plant (*Ibervillea sonorae*- Cucurbitaceae) has been employed medicinally by various ethnic groups in Northwestern Mexico for many centuries. Other common names include *Guereque* and *Guareque*. Early European explorers in Mexico such as Ignatz Pffeferkorn, for example, learned of this plant's antiseptic action on the skin, from various natives of the states of Sinaloa and Sonora (Weidauer and Rojas 2002; Vázquez 1999).

Wereke's application for the treatment of diabetes appears to be more recent, although little information exists as to the extent of time it has been employed internally as a hypoglycemic agent by Mexican traditional herbalists, especially in the States of Chihuahua, Nuevo León, Sinaloa and Sonora (Johnson et al., 1996).

In Ciudad Juarez, Chihuahua, for example, the root is commonly used and currently available in a variety of forms, such as the crude drug, liquid extracts and capsules, for example.

The medicinal use of this plant seems to be more localized in the North and Northwestern areas of Mexico (Vázquez, 1999; Johnson et al., 1996), as this plant is not commonly mentioned in publications from the southern or northeastern regions of that country (Adame and Adame, 2000; Aguilar, 1999; Gispert and Rodriguez, 1998; González, 1998; Linares et al., 1994; Martinez, 1989).

There is no information presently available that states whether Wereke does in fact contain any active ingredient (s) with hypoglycemic action similar to those found in other gourds belonging to the same botanical family (Cucurbitaceae) such as "bitter melon" (*Momordica charantia*), which is also used in Mexico as well as many other countries for the treatment of diabetes mellitus (Khare, 2003; Prajapati et al., 2003; Williamson, 2002; Parotta, 2002; Aguilar, 1999).

In Mexican traditional medicine, the dried root is pulverized and applied externally as a topical antiseptic for minor skin infections. The fresh root is sliced and applied to the skin, as a poultice, against arthritis and rheumatism (Aguilar, 1999; Argueta, 1994; Johnson et al., 1994). The root is employed as a decoction against diabetes, by boiling fragments of the root in water and ingesting it as tea. Wereke root is also available in capsules and extracts, although its effectiveness against diabetes has not been clinically evaluated.

There have been no toxicological evaluations of the plant, although, empirically, it is known to possess an abortifacient action (Weidauer and Rojas, 2002). For this reason, Wereke should never be used internally, in any form, during pregnancy and lactation.

No studies have ever been undertaken regarding its possible interactions with conventional drugs, especially oral hypoglycemics.

Yellow Oleander

Throughout Mexico and various other countries in Latin America, this plant (*Thevetia* spp.) is commonly known as: *Codo de Fraile*, *Yóyotl* , *Yoyote* (literally "rattle"), *Ayoyote, Alcanfura, Came, Cabalonga de la Huasteca, Hueso de Fraile, Solimán, Venenillo, Semilla del Brasil* and *Almendra quema-grasa* ("fat –burning almond").

This attractive ornamental shrub or medium-sized has bright yellow-orange flowers and milky latex. The plant belongs to the botanical family Apocynaceae and is originally from tropical America, but is now cultivated in many tropical and subtropical areas around the world. (Wagstaff, 2008).

Yellow oleander (*Thevetia neriifolia*) produces seeds which are highly poisonous and contain three glycosides--thevetin, thevetoxin and peruvoside. Clinical manifestations of poisoning range from mild to potentially fatal. The toxic glycosides have significant cardiovascular effects with varying rhythm abnormalities (Bose et al., 1999).

All parts of these plants are toxic (especially the seeds), and contain a variety of cardiac glycosides including thevetins A and B. Ingestion of yellow oleander results in nausea, vomiting, abdominal pain, diarrhea, cardiac dysrhythmias, and hyperkalemia (Bandara et al., 2010).

Although the plant is poisonous, yellow oleander has been used in Mexican traditional medicine for various health complaints, including its use (seed), as a charm against the "evil eye" and fallen fontanel in babies. A poultice made from the leaves has been applied externally to cure hemorrhoids, and the milky latex has been applied typically as a skin antiseptic; undoubtedly, a risky practice (Martinez, 1989).

Recently, the seed has been commercialized by some stores, as well as on the internet, as a "safe" and "natural" treatment for obesity. In various parts of Mexico, there have been numerous cases of intoxication with this herbal product which has been sold as capsules under diverse commercial names. The intoxicated individuals complained of vomiting, diarrhea, numbness of the extremities, intense abdominal pain, headaches, and dehydration. This situation prompted the Mexican federal pharmacovigilance authorities, known by the acronym COFEPRIS, to ban its use and confiscate thousands of seeds and capsules, but not with total success, as the product is still available under various commercial names on the internet (López- Villafranco and Camacho- Lacroix, 2002).

Various herbal or herbal/mineral combinations used in traditional medicine are currently being used around the world as therapeutic remedies for common ailments. Commonly known cardiotoxic herbs, such as *Thevetia peruviana* (yellow oleander), for example, may be included in diverse therapeutic preparations.

People intoxicated with these so-called weight loss products usually develop related symptoms, such as feelings of discomfort, nausea, dizziness, chest discomfort, and ventricular arrhythmias. Under these circumstances, it is of great importance that people seek proper medical attention and discontinue the use of the herbal preparation. Unfortunately, those individuals who believe that any herbal remedy is always safe are prone to be intoxicated if they self medicate with this herbal product (Dwivedi et al., 2011)

As stated previously, are no controlled clinical studies that confirm that yellow oleander seed can help reduce weight. On the other hand, there are various publications from around the world which confirm its significant toxicity to both humans and animals. For this reason, no part of the plant should ever be ingested, in any quantity.

Conclusion

Although the vegetable kingdom is definitely a source of important medicinal products, certain plants should be avoided due to their potential toxicity. Unfortunately, the lack of information regarding their negative effects, as well as the inadequate regulation of some of these products may result in serious and even fatal intoxications.

References

Adame J, Adame H. *Plantas Curativas del Noreste Mexicano*. Monterrey, Mexico: Ediciones Castillo; 2000.

Aguilar A. *Plantas Medicinales del Centro de México*. City: Guías Prácticas México Desconocido; 1999.

Argueta A. *Atlas de las Plantas de la Medicina Tradicional Mexicana. 3 Vols*. Mexico City: Instituto Nacional Indigenista; 1994.

Bandara V, Weinstein SA, White J, Eddleston M. A *review of the natural history, toxinology, diagnosis and clinical management of Nerium oleander (common oleander) and Thevetia peruviana (yellow oleander) poisoning. Toxicon.,* 56(3):273-81; 2010.

Bose TK, Basu RK, Biswas B, De JN, Majumdar BC, Datta S. Cardiovascular effects of yellow oleander ingestion. J Indian Med Assoc., 97(10):407-10; 1999.

Dickinson A. *History and overview of DSHEA.* Fitoterapia.: 82(1):5-10; 2011.

Dwivedi S, Aggarwal A, Sharma V. Cardiotoxicity from 'safe' herbomineral formulations. *Trop Doct.* ;41(2):113-5; 2011.

Gispert M and Rodriguez H. Los Coras*: Plantas Alimenticias y Medicinales De Su Ambiente Natural.* Mexico City: CONACULTA; 1998.

González M. *Plantas Medicinales del Noreste de México.* Monterrey, Mexico: IMSS-Vitro; 1998.

González-Stuart, A, Rivera J. *Comparison of Herbal Product Use in the Two Largest Border Communities between the US and Mexico Issue*: *HerbalGram* (81); 58-65; 2009.

Hocking G. A *Dictionary of Natural Products.* Medford, NJ: Plexus; 1997; p 30.

Johnson D, Moreno S and Lopez R. *Compendio Fitoquímico de La Medicina Tradicional Herbolaria de Sonora.* Hermosillo: Universidad de Sonora; 1996.

Khare C P. *Indian Herbal Remedies.* Berlin: Springer-Verlag; 2003.

Linares E, Flores B, Bye R. *Selección de Plantas Medicinales de México.* Mexico City: Limusa; 1994.

Locher CP, Burch MT, Mower HF, et al. Anti-microbial *activity and anti-complement activity of extracts obtained from selected Hawaiian medicinal plants.* J Ethnopharmacol. , 49(1):23-32; 1995.

López- Villafranco, M., Camacho- Lacroix, F. *Cuidado con el Codo de Fraile Abril 25 de 2002* http://gaceta.iztacala.unam.mx/187.pdf (accessed 5- 27-11).

Martinez M. *Las Plantas Medicinales de México.* Mexico City: Editorial Botas; 1989.

Nelson L, Shih R, Balick M. *Handbook of Poisonous and Injurious Plants*, 2nd ed. New York: Springer-Verlag; 2007; pp. 70-71.

Ostraff M, Anitoni K, Nicholson A, Booth GM. (2000). *Traditional Tongan cures for morning sickness and their mutagenic/toxicological evaluations.* J Ethnopharmacol.; 71(1-2):201-9.

Pamplona DDN. *Una mujer intoxicada por consumir "nuez de la india", una semilla para adelgazar.* Diario de Navarra- 3 de mayo de 2007 -http://www.diariodenavarra.es/actualidad/noticia.asp?not=2007050302105991&dia=20070503&seccion=navarra&seccion2=sucesos (accessed 5-27-11)

Parotta, J. *Healing Plants of Peninsular India.* London: Oxford University Press; 2002.

Pedrosa RC, Meyre-Silva C, Cechinel-Filho V, et al. *Hypolipidaemic activity of methanol extract of Aleurites moluccana.* Phytother Res. 2002 ; 16(8):765-8.

Prajapati N, Purohit S, Sharma A and Kumar T *Handbook of Medicinal Plants.* New Delhi: Agrobios - India; 2003.

Vázquez, R *Plantas Medicinales del Noroeste de México.* Mexico City: Guías México Desconocido # 4; 1999.

Wagstaff J. *International Poisonous Plant Checklist: An Evidence-Based Reference.* Boca Raton, FL: CRC Press; 2008:. 15.

Weidauer H and Rojas P. *Wereke - monografía.* Mexico City: Tlahui – Medic 2 (14); 2002.

Williamson E. *Major Herbs of Ayurveda.* London: Churchill- Livingstone.; 2002.

In: Vegetable Consumption and Health: New Research
Editors: Claudia Wilson and Melinda Morree
ISBN: 978-1-62100-941-2

Chapter 10

VEGETABLE CONSUMPTION BY OLDER ADULTS IN JAPAN

Andy H. Lee[1,*] and Fumi Hirayama[1,2]
[1]School of Public Health, Curtin Health Innovation Research Institute,
Curtin University, Perth, WA, Australia
Department of Global Health Policy, Graduate School of Medicine,
University of Tokyo, Tokyo, Japan

ABSTRACT

Background: The importance and health benefits of vegetables are well known, while the nutritional requirements of older adults are different from those of younger adults.

Objective: This study investigated vegetable consumption by gender and age groups among Japanese older adults.

Method: A total of 558 eligible participants (341 men and 217 women) aged 55 to 75 years were recruited from 10 districts/prefectures in middle and southern Japan. Information on habitual vegetable consumption was obtained by face-to-face interviews using a validated and reliable food frequency questionnaire.

Results: Women were found to consume more vegetables (mean 274, SD 166 g/day) than men (mean 207, SD 135 g/day) overall ($p < 0.001$) and across age groups 55-59, 60-64, 65-69 and 70-75 years. However, the intake levels of both genders did not vary significantly between age groups. The Japanese government has recommended an intake level of 350g or more per day for individuals. It is alarming that 83% of participants did not eat an adequate amount of vegetables.

Conclusion: Japanese older adults especially men should be encouraged to increase their vegetable consumption in order to maintain their health and well-being.

* Corresponding author: Professor Andy H. Lee, School of Public Health. Curtin University. GPO Box U 1987. Perth, WA, 6845, Australia. Phone: +61 8 92664180. Fax: +61 8 92662958. Email: Andy.Lee@curtin.edu.au.

INTRODUCTION

It is well known that diets high in vegetables are associated with lower rates of chronic diseases and cancers [1]. Vegetables provide a good source of nutrients and dietary fibre which are essential for various bodily functions. Throughout the world, reported vegetable consumptions are well below the recommended levels set by the World Health Organization [2], particularly for older adults. In the USA, for example, about one-third of adults aged 65 years and above consume vegetables three or more times a day [3]. In Australia, even after extensive social marketing campaigns promoting vegetable consumption, only 16% of older adults meet the recommended consumption level of five servings per day [4].

Japan has the third longest life expectancy in the world [5]. Its aging population (65 years and above) has been increasing rapidly from 7.9% in 1975 to 23.1% in 2010 [6]. Besides financial burden on the economy such as public pension and health care costs, the problems of social isolation and depression encountered by the Japanese elderly are major public health issues [7].

There is little information concerning vegetable consumption by Japanese older adults. The Japanese government has recommended eating 350g per day of vegetables for individuals [8], but there is no specific guideline available for older adults aged 65 years and above. The purpose of this report is to provide the latest update on habitual vegetable consumption by Japanese older adults. The findings have important implications for education, intervention and health promotion in Japan.

SUBJECTS AND METHODS

Study Design and Participants

Six hundred community-dwelling adults, aged between 55 and 75 years and residing in middle and southern Japan, were recruited into our cross-sectional study. Convenience sampling method was used in the recruitment of subjects. Participants were interviewed about habitual vegetable consumption when they visited shopping malls, attended community centers or undertook health checks at hospitals. Subjects were excluded if they experienced a recent stroke, dementia or had other health conditions that prohibited them from answering the questions. A total of 558 eligible participants from ten districts/prefectures (Tokyo, Aichi, Gifu, Kyoto, Shiga, Toyama, Niigata, Fukuoka, Nagasaki and Kumamoto) were available for analysis, after further excluding subjects with missing demographic details. Approval of the study protocol was obtained from the Human Research Ethics Committee of Curtin University.

Interview

A structured questionnaire was administered to collect demographic information, lifestyle characteristics, smoking and alcohol drinking status. All interviews were conducted face-to-face by the second author. The purpose of the study was explained to each participant before obtaining their written consent. Confidentiality of the information provided, and the right to withdraw without prejudice, were ensured and maintained throughout the study. The interviews, averaging 30 minutes in duration, took place in community centers, hospital outpatient departments, or local shopping malls.

Food Frequency Questionnaire

Information on habitual vegetable consumption was obtained using a 138-item food frequency questionnaire developed by the Japan Epidemiological Association [9]. This validated and reliable questionnaire asked about the usual consumption of 30 vegetables. The vegetable items included six pickled vegetables (Chinese radish, green leaf vegetable, plum, Chinese cabbage, cucumber, eggplant), seven cruciferous vegetables (cabbage, Chinese radish, komatsuna, broccoli, Chinese cabbage, leaf mustard, chard or Swiss chard), six green leafy vegetables (spinach, Chinese chive, garland chrysanthemum, bok choi, mugwort, green pepper), four yellow vegetables (carrot, tomato, pumpkin, tomato juice), and seven other vegetables (onion, cucumber, bean sprout, snap bean, lettuce, bitter gourd, loofah). The frequency of intake of vegetables was classified by nine categories: 'almost never', 'once to three times per month', 'once to twice per week', 'three to four times per week', 'five to six times per week', 'once per day', 'twice to three times per day', 'four to six times per day', and 'seven or more times per day'. Standard portion size was specified for each item, with three choices of amount: small (50% smaller), medium (same as the standard), and large (50% larger). The total amount of vegetables consumed (in grams) per day was calculated from summing the responses recorded.

Statistical Analysis

Descriptive statistics were used to summarize the characteristics of participants. Univariate tests (chi-square, *t* test and ANOVA) were applied to compare vegetable consumption levels between genders and age groups (55-59, 60-64, 65-69, 70-75 years). All statistical analyses were undertaken using the SPSS for Windows package version 15.

RESULTS

The majority of the 558 eligible participants were men (61%) with mean age 63.3 (SD 6.2) years and mean body mass index 23.4 (SD 3.1) kg/m^2. Most of them (79%) were married and had attained high school education (63%). A substantial proportion of participants was current smokers (18%) and drank alcohol regularly (60%). About 38% of them were pensioners or had completely retired from the work force. The prevalence of chronic illnesses (such as hypertension, diabetes, cardiovascular disease) was 49% in this sample. Overall, the vegetable intake level was significantly lower among males (mean 207, SD 135 g/day) than their female counterparts (mean 274, SD 166 g/day), $p < 0.001$. Table 1 shows their habitual vegetable consumption by gender and age group. The lower consumption levels of the male participants were evident at each age group ($p < 0.05$). However, there were no significant differences across age groups overall ($p = 0.06$) and separately for men ($p = 0.44$) and women ($p = 0.07$).

Table 1. Vegetable consumption levels (g/day) of Japanese older adults by gender and age group

Age group (years)	Male (n = 341)		Female (n = 217)		Both gender (n = 558)	
	mean	SD	mean	SD	mean	SD
55-59	199	(126)	244	(150)	215	(136)
60-64	212	(141)	302	(156)	243	(152)
65-69	228	(165)	321	(235)	262	(198)
70-75	194	(108)	263	(134)	229	(126)
Overall	207	(135)	274	(166)	233	(151)

Table 2. Prevalence of inadequate vegetable intake (< 350 g/day) of Japanese older adults by gender and age group

Age group (years)	Male (n = 341)	Female (n = 217)	Both gender (n = 558)
55-59	89.1%	76.3%	84.5%
60-64	87.5%	71.4%	82.0%
65-69	86.2%	68.4%	79.6%
70-75	89.8%	80.3%	85.0%
Overall	88.3%	75.1%	83.2%

We next compare the vegetable intake level of each individual with the Japanese government's recommendation of 350g per day. Table 2 gives the prevalence of inadequate vegetable intake by gender and age group. The prevalence of inadequacy was high, ranging from 68.4% among women aged 65-69 years to almost 90% for elderly men aged 70 years and above. Overall, the problem of inadequate intake was more prevalent among men (88.3%) than women (75.1%), $p < 0.001$.

DISCUSSION

This study investigated habitual vegetable consumption of Japanese adults aged 55 to 75 years with respect to gender and age group. The observed intake levels were comparable with those reported in a population-based survey conducted by the Japanese Ministry of Health, Labour and Welfare [10], even though the sampling method and age range used were different. Both sets of results indicated the substantially lower vegetable consumption by older men. The overall mean intake of our participants was also relatively low at 233 (SD 151) g/day, with the majority not achieving the daily recommended level of 350g set by the Japanese government [8]. It is alarming that only 17% of older adults exceeded this target.

The finding appears to be consistent with other countries. For example, only a mere 6% of Americans aged over 60 years met the recommendation of three servings of vegetables per day [11], while 16% of older Australians attained the recommended five servings or 375g per day [4].

The nutritional requirements of older adults are different from those of younger adults [1]. Eating adequate amounts of vegetables can provide essential nutrients to bolster the immune system and protect against chronic diseases, as well as minimizing the adverse physiological changes associated with ageing [12]. Recognizing the differences in requirement between age groups, appropriate dietary guidelines and recommended intake levels should be developed for older adults, especially for Japanese aged over 65 years, in order to maintain their health and well-being.

In this study, detailed information on habitual vegetable consumption was obtained by self- report using a validated and reliable instrument. As with other surveys of elderly subjects, the responses from our participants inevitably incurred some recall error due to possible memory and cognitive loss. Therefore, face-to-face interviews were used to increase the response rate and to improve the accuracy of their answers. All interviews were conducted by the same investigator (second author) to minimize any potential misinterpretation of the questions and to eliminate interviewer bias. However, individual consumption pattern can vary by season, resulting in some bias when estimating their frequencies of habitual intake.

A limitation of our study was the lack of qualitative data on the perception and attitude of the older adults in relation to their vegetable intake. Their opinion and consumption behaviour were not solicited due to time constraints. Another limitation concerned the adequacy of our convenience sample, which consisted of voluntary participants recruited from community centers, shopping malls and outpatient clinics. Although systematic bias was unlikely and little heterogeneity in vegetable consumption was found across prefectures and data collection sites, further replications and using food dairy records are recommended to confirm the generalizability of the findings.

In conclusion, Japanese older adults, especially elderly men, should be targeted by the government for education and health promotion programs to increase their vegetable consumption. As the aging population increases there is an urgent need to develop sound interventions capable of making a positive behavioral change for older adults.

REFERENCES

[1] National Health and Medical Research Council. *Dietary Guidelines for Older Australians.* Government Publishing Service, Canberra, Australia, 1999.

[2] Baker AH, Wardle J. Sex differences in fruit and vegetable intake in older adults. *Appetite*, 2003; 40 (3), 269-275.

[3] Blanck HM, Gillespie C, Kimmons JE, Seymour JD, Serdula MK. Trends in fruit and vegetable consumption among U.S. men and women, 1994-2005. *Preventing Chronic Disease*, 2008; 5 (2), 1-10.

[4] Daly A, Roberts L. Collaborative Health and Wellbeing Survey and 2002 *Health and Wellbeing Surveillance System: Eating, Exercise and Body Size in Western Australian Populations*. Department of Health, Western Australia, 2000.

[5] Central Intelligence Agency. Rank Order - Life Expectancy at Birth. https://www.cia.gov/library/publications/the-world-factbook/rankorder/2102rank.html.
[6] Ministry of Internal Affairs and Communications. Statistics Bureau of Japan. http://www.stat.go.jp/data/jinsui/pdf/201103.pdf.
[7] Okumura R. "Idea of cohabitation" in aging society - local cohobitation of aging baby boomers - Part 1: aging society in 2005. Mitsubishi Sogo Kenkyujo Syoho, 2005; 45: 60-73.
[8] Japanese Ministry of Health, Labour and Welfare. Health Japan 21. http://www1.mhlw.go.jp/topics/kenko21_11/top.html.
[9] Japan Epidemiological Association. Validity and reproducibility of self-administered food frequency questionnaires in the Japan public health center-based prospective study on cancer and cardiovascular diseases (JPHC Study). *Journal of Epidemiology*, 2003; 13 (1 suppl): s148-s162.
[10] Japanese Ministry of Health, Labour and Welfare. Health and Nutrition Survey for Japanese in 2009. http://www.mhlw.go.jp/houdou/2008/12/h1225-5a.html.
[11] Jarvis KL, Friedman RH, Heeren T, Cullinane PM. Older women and physical activity: using the telephone to walk. *Women's Health Issues*, 1997, 7 (1): 24 -29.
[12] Carter P, Gray LJ, Troughton J, Khunti K, Davies MJ. Fruit and vegetable intake and incidence of type 2 diabetes mellitus: systematic review and meta-analysis. *British Medical Journal*, 2010, 341: c4229.

INDEX

A

B

C

D

G

H

M

N

Q

R

S

T

U

V

W

X

Y

Z